EATING TO LIVE™
UNLOCKING THE LEAKY GUT CODE

Tiffany!
Good luck on your
Journey to Optimal
Health!
Love you! Carla

EATING TO LIVE™
UNLOCKING
THE LEAKY GUT CODE

A Customized Journey to Optimal Health

By

David and Carla Meine, CFNC

With Kristin McQuivey

ISBN: 978-1-7374382-0-5 (Paperback)

Library of Congress Control Number: 2021914323

Statements in this book have not been evaluated by the Food and Drug Administration. Products are not intended to diagnose, treat, cure or prevent any disease. If you are pregnant, nursing, taking medication, or have a medical condition, consult your physician before using our products. You should not stop taking any medication without first consulting your physician. The information provided here is for informational and educational purposes only and is not intended as medical advice or a substitute for advice from your physician or other qualified healthcare professional. You should not use the information for diagnosis or treatment of any health problem or for prescription of any medication or other treatment. ALWAYS consult with a healthcare professional before starting any diet, exercise program, or dietary supplements.

Book design by Author Your Brand.

First printing edition 2021.

Eating to Live Publishing
2701 N. Thanksgiving Way, Suite 100
Lehi, UT, 84043
www.eatingtolive.com

TABLE OF CONTENTS

Part I 9

Prologue. How It All Began 11

Chapter 1. "You Have Cancer" 15

Chapter 2. Anything but Chemotherapy 29

Chapter 3. Frankenstein's Office 43

Chapter 4. A Little Hope Is a Powerful Thing 55

Chapter 5. A Sidestep into Foot Problems 63

Chapter 6. ADHD: My Superpower 73

Chapter 7. The Third Time's a Charm 83

Chapter 8. Oh NO! Not Sleep Apnea, Too! 99

Chapter 9. 61 Years Old and Falling Apart (My Dependence on NSAIDs) 113

Chapter 10. Healing My Leaky Gut 129

Chapter 11. Connecting the Dots 139

Chapter 12. Meeting Dr. Gundry: The Legendary Physician of Restorative Medicine 153

Chapter 13. The Last Dot Revealed: Visceral Fat 165

Chapter 14. My Ongoing Battle with My Greatest Nemesis: Sugar 177

Level Up: Part 2 of Eating to Live 191

Level 1 203

Chapter 1. An Introduction to Level 1 205

Chapter 2. Finding Your WHY to Achieving Your Optimal Health 221

Chapter 3. The Eating to Live Journal 243

Chapter 4. The Eating to Live Meal Plan 247

Chapter 5. Drink More Water 255

LEVEL 2 269
Chapter 1. An Introduction to Level 2. 271
Chapter 2. Get Plenty of Sleep. 279
Chapter 3. Remove NSAIDs from Your Diet 295

LEVEL 3 307
Chapter 1. An Introduction to Level 3. 309
Chapter 2. Train Your Brain for Optimal Health 319
Chapter 3. Supplement Your Food with Proper Nutrition 339

LEVEL 4 353
Chapter 1. An Introduction to Level 4 355
Chapter 2. Reduce Stress. 363
Chapter 3. Exercise for a Healthy Body. 377

Conclusion 389
Epilogue. 391
Appendix I. 397

Dear Readers,

We realize that memories are imperfect and individual, but the story we share here is ours, and we have shared it to the very best of our mutual recollection. We hope that by sharing it we are able to help you on your own individual journey toward achieving optimal health.

With love,
David and Carla Meine

PART I

PROLOGUE

HOW IT ALL BEGAN

Shortly after 9/11, I came across Carla's profile on an internet dating site. I read about her passion for sports, travel, camping, and her deep love for her family. Many of our hobbies and interests were a perfect match, and we had similar experience in business as well. I knew I wanted to meet this woman. Because of her busy dating schedule, I couldn't secure a date with her until November 9th. In the meantime, we started talking on the phone and quickly developed a fun, comfortable banter. I found myself really looking forward to that November date.

One perfect date later, we spent every minute we could together from then on. When we weren't together, we were on the phone with each other. I proposed less than two months later on January 2nd, and we were married January 17th.

Neither of our families were thrilled. They were worried things had happened too quickly. We could certainly understand why they thought that, but when you know, you know!

A few months later, I ended up joining the company Carla had founded, with the responsibility to grow the business and get it sold. Carla and I discovered that we not only made a great team in our marriage, but we made great partners in business as well. I was thoroughly enjoying my new role in her company, and our strengths really complemented each other.

Prior to working together, I had spent significant time traveling for business. It seemed I was constantly battling some sort of health issue or another. I had been diagnosed with colitis and then Crohn's disease in the 1980s. I was also frequently sick with flu, bronchitis, or pneumonia. I thought it was because of the stress on my system from all the non-stop travel and the unhealthy, recycled airplane air I was forced to breathe. I also had a lot of pain from old sports injuries. It was frustrating to have life constantly interrupted with health issues, and even more so because I was a competitive athlete. Back then, I was training twenty-two to twenty-four hours per week to get ready for the Ironman® race that June. Carla started riding or running with me just so we could spend more time together. It never occurred to me that she would also get hooked on the sport.

I started researching nutrition information so that I could stay healthier and perform at an optimal level. The nutraceutical world was so confusing! Each supplement made various claims, but ultimately said they provided a missing ingredient in our diets that was necessary for optimal health. So, I did the easy thing: I just started taking them all. Needless to say, my troublesome health struggles continued, despite the fact that I was in good shape and still competing athletically.

In 2003, Carla and I developed a successful business that helped others to lose weight and get into shape by following sound nutritional principles. We have since sold that business with the intention of retiring and focusing on our family, but it has become our passion to share what we've learned and help others improve their quality of life.

Throughout these years, I lived what I thought was a healthy lifestyle and had a robust team of doctors for every ailment, but my problems and pain persisted and even escalated into life-and-death battles. Carla and I became dedicated to finding answers. We wanted not just to survive, but thrive, and grow old together.

So began our journey to true optimal health. It wasn't easy. It took persistence and some long-suffering. It took lots of trial and error, too. Looking back over the past seventeen years, I can see the beginnings of our education in the world of nutrition, vitality, and health. Each small step along the journey has helped us learn life-changing and life-saving lessons; each discovery an important piece of the puzzle. We share our story with you in the hope that you, too, will discover optimal health, and join with us in our adventure to wellness through "eating to live."

CHAPTER 1

"YOU HAVE CANCER"

The room was dark, and the buzzing light from the fluorescent bulbs in the hallway glinted off the steel handrail of my hospital bed. The elastic band of the powder blue cap covering my head itched, and I pulled at it as I shifted, trying to alleviate the pain in my back. Over the past years, intense back pain had become a daily part of my life. During these excruciating months, I had attempted to alleviate this debilitating pain through years of chiropractic visits, acupuncture, flotation tanks, upside-down back therapy, pain medication, and physical therapy, but every potential remedy failed. So now I was about to do what I'd worked so hard to avoid. This invasive and risky surgery was our last resort to try and mitigate the physically-limiting agony my back caused every day.

Pain in various forms was not new to me, and I didn't consider myself part of the "man-cold" group; I was more in the "push-through-the-pain" club. I had been a competitive amateur athlete all of my life. Football, wrestling, track, basketball, softball—I loved it all. In my twenties, I competed in cycling. Depending on the season, I spent every spare moment water skiing, snowboarding, or snow skiing. Then in my forties, I got caught up in being a triathlete and competed all over the United States in forty-two Olympic-distance events. I even completed an Ironman® race. I loved the adrenaline of it all, but my body did not survive unscathed.

Because of injuries incurred during these years, I switched to competitive tennis in my fifties. Carla—my wife and partner in everything I did—and I took the bronze medal at the Senior National Tournament, which is pretty much the Olympics for people over fifty. After more injuries, we switched to pickleball, where I was no less competitive with a smaller racquet and plastic Wiffle Ball. We started winning gold and silver medals in competitive pickleball tournaments, even qualifying in 2018 to play in the US National Pickleball Tournament in Palm Springs.

Now in my sixties, I was paying a heavy price for all those years of intense activity. Over the past four decades, many over-the-counter painkillers had been part of my daily routine. It was very common for me to take 800 mgs of Ibuprofen three times a day. When that was no longer enough, doctors prescribed Lortab or Naproxen. This back pain, however, was a whole new level of suffering. I couldn't just throw back a handful of Advil and grit my teeth through it anymore. For the past few years, I'd have episodes where I'd bend down to pick up a piece of lint from the carpet, and my back would spasm. I'd fall down in excruciating pain, unable to get back up. Eventually, I'd crawl across the house to my bedroom, where my wife—bless her—would get underneath me and basically squat me into the bed, where I'd remain for the next three days.

I'd spent three years with a chiropractor, who assured me he could absolutely fix my back. Turns out, he absolutely couldn't.

So, I started working with my good friend from college instead. Rogan Taylor is a Doctor of Physical Therapy and was very confident from the beginning that he could solve my problem without invasive surgery. I spent three afternoons a week for the next two years in his office receiving an uncomfortable treatment I had snippily dubbed "wet table electroshock therapy." I would have tolerated it better had it been helping, but the intense back pain remained constant.

"Hey, Rogan," I finally said. "You have been working on me for two years now, and this agonizing pain is getting worse."

My good friend leaned back against the counter and looked at me quietly for a few moments. "David, we gave it everything we have. I think it's time you talk to a surgeon. I'm sorry, bud."

He knew that wasn't what I wanted to hear, but it had now been five years of severe pain. I sighed, looked down at the floor, and nodded in defeat.

The earliest date available for surgery was six months out, in February. I didn't know how I'd survive the pain until then. I was barely able to walk. And it was affecting my ability to work. I'd recently hosted our company's annual customer event, but when we pulled up to the restaurant, I couldn't get out of the car and walk in. I tried and tried to pull myself up to standing, leaning on Carla, beads of sweat peppering my forehead from the effort. To my utter mortification, I couldn't do it. Even with the Lortab pain medication I was on, I couldn't walk the few feet from my car to the restaurant. Fortunately, they had a wheelchair, and Carla was able to wheel me in and up to my spot in the front of the room. Somehow, I coped through the dinner and my speech, but it felt so humiliating. This was a definite low point for me.

Many phone calls later, I was able to get the surgery moved up to October. Although I was still so discouraged about needing such an invasive surgery, I was immensely grateful and immediately accepted. As we prepared for the surgery, concerns repeatedly rattled me. At the time, I had nine grandchildren, and I hated the thought of not being able to be a hands-on grandpa. I also worried about being able to maintain a demanding work schedule with a company where so many were counting on me.

Meanwhile, my wife was having different thoughts. Let me back up here a moment and introduce you to her: Carla and I have now been married for eighteen years. We have a blended family of seven kids and eighteen grandchildren—wonderful chaos! Carla was by my side, not just as a cheerleader, but as a fierce competitor and teammate for every triathlon, race, and tournament. She is an avid snow skier and cycler, and she can surf behind a boat with the best of them. She is also my business partner, and our strengths and work ethic complement each other in a strong and equal partnership. This back issue was a real challenge for our relationship, because we went from being super active and on-the-go nonstop to... nothing. We'd been told this would be an extra-difficult surgery, and that I would be completely down for two months afterwards and unable to do much at all for a full six months. Looking back now, we both wish it had been so easy!

Carla is a remarkable force for good who is able to remain positive despite hard challenges. She had been with me through a few other surgeries and knew I never reacted well to anesthesia. Her worried thoughts included, "How long until we will be able to resume our normal lives again?" And, "*Will* we be able to resume normal life again?"

It's a good thing we didn't know how long it would take to get back to "normal." The surgery was brutal. Recovery was grueling. What they said would take four to six months took me a year. But before then, things got much worse.

I imagine you might be asking yourself, "What does all this back stuff have to do with cancer?" Three months after that surgery, I started having a strange symptom that I thought was related to my back surgery. Around the end of January, I had this weird thing happen when I urinated. There appeared to be a significant amount of blood in my urine. The bright red color was shocking. What was happening? In my ignorance, I thought it seemed like something that would only happen to women on a monthly basis. I didn't understand it and was embarrassed to discuss it with anyone, including my wife. It didn't happen again the next day, though, and I forgot about it.

It happened again in February, just once, and again I didn't tell anyone about it. In March, it started happening about once a week, but I really thought it stemmed from my surgery and would go away as my back healed. Then it returned at the beginning of April. For three straight days, I'd stare into the toilet bowl each time I went and see all of the bright red blood. I was officially scared.

For some reason, I thought providing a sample would be important. Never one to do anything halfway, I grabbed an empty quart-sized jar from our food storage and filled the whole thing up. It was sitting on the bathroom counter when Carla walked in. I pointed to it—not that she'd be able to miss the shocking specimen.

"Hey honey," I asked her. "Um... Do you think I need to be worried about that?"

Don't ask me why, after three months of hiding my problem in complete embarrassment, I chose to shock her now with this extreme visual version of my problem. I'll never forget the look on her face.

"Oh my gosh, David!" she exclaimed, horrified. "You have blood in your urine?! You've got to get to the doctor right now! This is not something you mess around with!" She insisted I drive down to Instacare immediately.

Even though I very considerately provided my full-jar specimen for them, shoved into a brown lunch snack and awkwardly hidden under my jacket, the Instacare doctor required a fresh sample. "Doc, what is going on here?" I asked the thin, balding doctor. What is this?" I gestured toward the full Mason jar.

"Well, we need to see if you have a bladder infection." He paused for a moment, then continued. "We'll test the urine sample that you're going to give us right now, and it'll be good news if you test positive for a bladder infection."

It didn't dawn on me until later what he'd really meant by that statement. I returned to the waiting room for the results. When they escorted me back again, this time the doctor looked at me very seriously. He still skipped the small talk, leading with, "It's bad news. You don't have a bladder infection." I then learned what a urologist was, and that I'd need to see one—the sooner the better.

Carla and I still weren't too worried—she really thought this was something like a UTI—and we were happy to see our good friend and neighbor Ron Oldroyd on the referral list of urologists. I called him with my situation, and he got me right in.

"What Did He Just Say?"

If I thought I was embarrassed about my discolored pee, all modesty now flew out the window. A cystoscopy exam is an extremely hands-on, thorough procedure. It's probably similar to what women have to go through all the time—feet in stirrups, any sense of privacy completely invaded—but this was all very new to me! I looked away and tried to take myself to my "happy place" while Dr. Oldroyd maneuvered the tiny camera on the end of the flexible tubing up through my urethra, past the prostate, and into my bladder. It's uncomfortable and messy, as the tube also shoots out water to keep things clean and expand the bladder, eliminating any possible folds. The water ran out and dripped down my butt, soaking the paper I was sitting on. It was hard to concentrate on the words he was saying, because all I could think was, *How much longer 'til he gets this thing out of me?*

He was peering intently at the screen, twisting the camera in awkward ways, trying to capture all angles. He adjusted his glasses further up his nose and started counting. "Oh yes, I can see there's one...two... There's another, so three... Three good-sized tumors. You have cancer, David."

What? I thought to myself. *What did he just say?*

"One of the tumors has a burst blood vessel, hence the blood in your urine. That's a miracle, really. Usually we don't catch tumors like this so early." He looked up, his face serious, his eyes meeting mine. "We won't know for sure until we can biopsy it, but I'm pretty sure they're cancerous." I was still stunned and trying to catch up with what he was saying. "We've got to get you right into surgery. As in, tomorrow."

I'm actually not certain of anything else he said. All my brain heard was, "You have cancer." It fixated there, stuck on those words as if in a deep, inescapable rut. In a blur, they scheduled me for emergency surgery first thing in the morning, and I left the office, shocked and emotional. Because we both thought this appointment really wasn't going to be any big deal, Carla had stayed home to get some work done. How was I going to tell her? I was still really struggling to recuperate from my back surgery. How could I possibly handle another one so soon?

Carla

As I heard the words David was saying, I was in shock. My initial reaction was, *No, that can't be right! That happens to other people, people who don't take care of themselves, who aren't healthy!* Even though you know that isn't really true—you know plenty of folks who were fit and took care of themselves who unfairly get cancer—but you just think, *This can't be happening to us.*

My thoughts came fast and furious, a rollercoaster of shock and denial and grief. In one brief moment, our life completely changed. This was going to change absolutely everything!

My typical response is to look for the good, so I naturally started saying, "Could be it's not cancer, David. We have to wait and see..." And then, "But if it is, we'll get through this. We have lots of friends and family who will pray for us."

I really wasn't sure how David was actually feeling, but I knew I'd need to stay strong for him. I didn't want us to start wallowing (as is so easy and understandable to do) in the "Why us? What did we do wrong to deserve this?" thought swamp. Instead, the problem solver in me took over. I started making mental lists.

Surgery at 5 a.m. tomorrow. What do we need to do? This is our lot, so let's get to work. What can we do? We needed to get ourselves ready as best we could. We both needed to clear our incredibly full schedules. Mentally, I ticked down the list of things we'd need to handle.

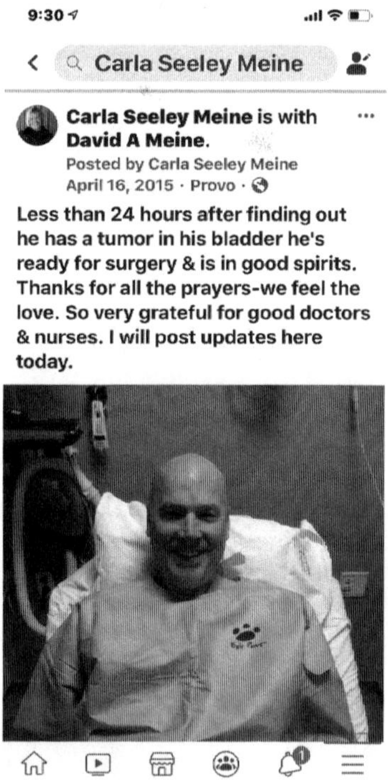

David and I hugged each other, and the tears flowed down my face. "We will get through this together, David." I felt the truth and peace of that statement with all my heart. "Whatever happens, we'll face it together." We then knelt together and prayed, petitioning God for His help and guidance through this. Our faith has been a source of strength to us many times in our life. As we prayed, I had the strongest impression that we needed to let all our friends and family know so they could pray for us, too. I told David, "We need to let all the family know. You call your kids, parents, and siblings. I'll call mine, and we need to let our friends know, too. I feel like all our friends would want to know and pray for you."

It can be hard and humbling to ask for help, but after calling our close friends and asking for their strength and prayers, David let me post on Facebook. He wasn't sure he was comfortable with that, but I convinced him we needed all our friends and anybody else who was willing to join us in prayer.

All of this was very emotional. But it was also very faith-promoting. The next day, as he went in for the procedure, instead of feeling anxious about him going under anesthesia again or about what the results would be, I felt an amazing sense of peace. I knew I was being buoyed up by all those prayers from all our loved ones.

Carla Seeley Meine ···
Posted by Carla Seeley Meine
April 15, 2015 · West Jordan ·

Friends we are asking for your prayers tonight. My hubby David has a tumor in his bladder that has to be removed. Thankfully our friend Ron Oldroyd got him right in & got him diagnosed & has scheduled him for surgery in the morning. We are feeling very blessed that it was discovered early & is treatable.

Carla Seeley Meine ···
Posted by Carla Seeley Meine
April 16, 2015 · Provo ·

Surgery went well. There were 3 tumors so we're really glad our doctor got him in right away. He's very optimistic that David will have a full recovery. Thanks again for all the prayers. We have felt them.

David

The outpouring of love from family and friends, and even people we barely knew, was amazing. Surgery went well. Dr. Oldroyd found the three tumors he'd spotted during the scope. One of them was large and had to be cut out of the lining of my bladder. "It's a good thing we caught this when we did," he told me from my bedside, post-op. "That was Stage T2a cancer. If that tumor had broken through the bladder wall, then you're known as the Walking Dead."

Gulp. Evidently bladder cancer is known as "transitional cancer." It's often just a matter of time before the cancer takes over your internal organs and you die. Most folks have no symptoms, and they don't find out until it's too late.

That "embarrassing symptom" that started back in January had saved my life. We truly believed we had received a miracle with that early symptom and such quick and competent treatment.

"The Cancer Is Back"

In July 2015, I went in for my three-month bladder scan. Dr. Oldroyd and I got up close and personal again with another fun cystoscopy exam. This time, however, he smiled and told me everything looked good. My bladder wall was healing nicely.

I rushed home to give Carla the good news. We texted and called all our family and friends who cheered. We had won! We'd caught the cancer early and there was nothing to worry about. We went about our lives as we always had, barely giving cancer another thought.

In December 2015, I returned for my next checkup. I sat in the waiting room chair, my legs bouncing with anticipation. *Let's get this over with,* I thought, full of optimism and ready to get back to my busy life. I looked around the room at the handful of other patients. An older gentleman was sitting across from me, talking with his daughter about his stage 4 prostate cancer. He sounded grim and looked tired. I sat there feeling so thankful I wasn't him.

When it was my turn, I joked around with Dr. Oldroyd. He'd had a heart procedure done the week after my bladder surgery, so I asked him how the ticker was and teased him about his cold hands. He was in a good mood, and we were laughing. By this third go-around, we were pretty darn comfortable with each other.

Suddenly he went quiet and started intently looking at the monitor. He started turning the knob, trying to get the flexible tubing to where he needed it to go. The look of concern on his face gave him away. My heart rate immediately spiked. *Please,* I thought to myself. *Don't tell me there are more tumors.*

I felt sick as he started counting. "One...two...three..." He was quiet for a moment, then, "I can see at least six. Six new tumors." I was frozen and remained speechless as he pulled the equipment out. "We need to get you into surgery right away, David. First thing in the morning, let's go get you scheduled."

I drove home completely stunned. The fifteen-minute drive seemed to take hours. I remember the stark, looming mountains covered in snow and the wind whipping around the car. The Christmas decorations and twinkling lights that usually symbolized joy and hope seemed an affront to the ugly knowledge that cancer had been growing silently, insidiously, inside me.

How had I gone from no tumors five months ago to six tumors—maybe more—so quickly? I'd finally gotten my life back! My back was finally feeling healed, and I'd gotten back into some of the hobbies I loved. Our company was still growing at over 200% for the second year in a row. Life was good! So why this? Why was this happening again to me, to my wife? I already dreaded having to tell Carla the terrible news.

I found her sitting on the floor, playing with one of our grandchildren. Smiling, she looked up at me and asked how the appointment went. When she saw my face, she immediately knew something was very wrong. After hesitating a moment, the words spilled out of me. "Dr. Oldroyd saw at least six new tumors. He wants me in surgery tomorrow morning."

"Oh no, this cannot be happening!" Carla started to cry, stood up, and gave me a long, fierce hug, supporting each other as we cried together.

Driving in the dark the next morning, all I could think about was a story my good friend had told me about his father who had struggled with bladder cancer. Somehow during the previous cystoscopy exam he'd had, the urologist missed a fold in the bladder where a tumor was hiding. He'd pronounced it clean of cancer. The next year, his father died of stage 4 cancer. The undetected tumor had gone through the bladder wall and attacked his organs. I was visualizing this happening inside of me and the thought made me physically ill. My friend had strongly recommended I have my bladder removed, but I did not want to have to use a urostomy pouch. "Please, God, let this surgery work!" I repeatedly prayed.

Getting prepped for surgery was like terrible déjá vu. As I laid in my hospital bed, the nurses were bustling around, and all of the commotion was making me anxious. When the anesthesiologist came over and asked if I was ready, I wanted to scream, "No!" Instead, I gave him a weak smile and said, "Yes." I realized that, this time, I was truly scared.

My next memory was of waking up in a fuzzy room. I tried to get my eyes to focus and looked around for my wife. I saw her in the chair near my bed and could see the relief on her face as our eyes met. "How many tumors did they find?" were the first words out of my mouth.

"Fourteen," she said. "But none of them penetrated the bladder wall." I sighed in relief and closed my eyes.

Carla Seeley Meine ···
Posted by Carla Seeley Meine
December 16, 2015 · Lindon ·

"The Cancer is Back" words you never want to hear but that's what the doctor told David today. His bladder cancer is back and so we're back in the hospital tomorrow morning for surgery. Then he starts Chemo in January. All the prayers really helped last time so we'd appreciate that again.

Carla Seeley Meine is with **David A Meine.** ···
Posted by Carla Seeley Meine
December 17, 2015 · Provo ·

Thanks again for all the sweet comments & prayers. Surgery went great. Doctor says they got all of them. (There were 14 but they were tiny so they got it early. He's in recovery. We'll be home late this afternoon.

CHAPTER 2

ANYTHING BUT CHEMOTHERAPY

The next voice I heard was that of Dr. Oldroyd. "How you doing, champ?" Without waiting for a response, he continued on. "So we found more than we thought in there, but once again you were lucky in that we got them out in time. However, if we find any tumors at your next checkup, I recommend you get started on some chemotherapy."

My eyes flew open and my whole body filled with stress and fear. Was he really telling me I might have more tumors in another three months? *Oh no,* I thought to myself. *Heck no. I absolutely have to find an alternative to chemotherapy! I am not doing that!*

I've known so many people who have struggled with some form of cancer. Many have endured chemo and radiation. In my mind, this is truly an example of a cure that is worse than the disease. I've heard horror stories of the side effects. Chemo kills the bad cells, but it also ends up killing vital good cells as well, like those in the bone marrow that help maintain our supply of important white blood cells. I'd heard about someone who got the flu after chemo and died because, due to a low white cell blood count, the body could not fight off the infection. Someone else's kidney got damaged during chemo, and they suffered greatly from that side effect.

For some reason, when you have your own struggle with cancer, you get to hear everyone's worst-case stories. There were also plenty of folks who seemed compelled to tell me about losing a loved one to cancer. These conversations provoked a deep uneasiness in me, down in my core. They had no idea of the anxiety they caused me.

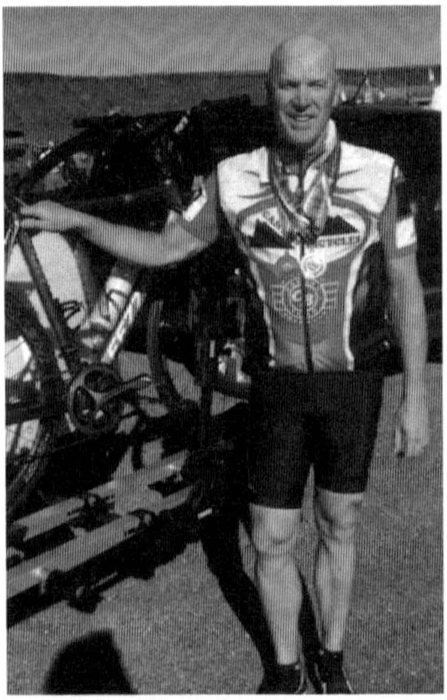

So, I did what I always do when presented with a problem: I got on the internet. Whenever I need to research answers and solve issues, I start with Google. Sitting at the computer I typed in all capital letters: BLADDER CANCER and NATUROPATHIC CURES. As I typed each letter, I hammered the keys with my fingers. I had officially entered the "angry" stage, and my keyboard was taking the brunt of it. *Why me?* I was fuming. I'd specifically made healthy choices all these years because of the bad examples I'd had in my life. My dad had smoked three packs of cigarettes a day since he'd been a teen and was an alcoholic. I hated it. When I was thirteen years old, he had me taste whiskey, and it made me sick. I made a commitment to myself that I would never drink alcohol or take drugs. I didn't even drink coffee. My one vice was Coca-Cola, and I even gave that up for two years during this cancer journey. Plus, I'd worked so hard to stay in top physical shape as an athlete. I looked at a framed picture on my desk that someone had snapped of me as I was finishing a triathlon.

How could the outside of my body be in such good shape while inside I was growing cancer tumors like crazy?

Even with all the research I was doing, I didn't connect certain dots. I'd struggled with another health problem during the past fifteen years that seemed completely unrelated. I had severe neuropathy in my feet (I talk about this in more detail in Chapter 5). The best description of this was that my feet felt like they were on fire. Our kitchen and master bedroom had marble floors, and I'd stand on them barefooted to minimize the pain. At night I'd make sure the sheets and blankets didn't touch my feet because it was so painful.

I also had very painful arthritis in my right knee, left hand, and throughout my spine and neck. Again, as a competitive athlete, my mantra was just to work through the pain, and it never occurred to me (or any of my doctors, either) that perhaps the neuropathy, back problems, and cancer were all related.

I also didn't connect this cancer experience with the various skin cancers I'd had. Since my early forties, my dermatologist had aggressively used his cryotherapy gun of liquid nitrogen to freeze off anything that looked suspicious, including some basal cell and squamous cell carcinomas. I'd spent many summers lifeguarding at Glenwood Springs, the world's largest outdoor hot springs pool and the coolest place ever for a teenage boy to work. What wasn't so cool was the awful sunburn I always got my first week there. The tops of my feet were so burned I got sun poisoning. The rest of the summer, I'd coat my skin in baby oil and let those rays bake right in. Back then, sunscreen wasn't a thing, and I definitely paid the price.

I never thought about all of these separate things as being related. I didn't clue into the possibility of having immune system issues at all. Thinking that I had been making healthy choices, it also never occurred to me that what I ate and drank could be weakening my ability to heal my body. I was truly "living to eat" in my forties and fifties. I didn't take into consideration any of these issues when looking for an alternative to chemotherapy for my bladder.

Carla and I began looking at many approaches. Each one had to be developed and managed by a doctor. We found a local Naturopathic Doctor in Provo, Utah. I really wanted to trust her experience and advice. One of the first steps she recommended was Vitamin C and D IVs once a week to boost my immune system. It was at this point of my cancer journey that I finally realized I was dealing with a compromised immune system.

It was all really humbling. During the weeks after my surgery, I was becoming an expert internet researcher. I was completely driven by the goal of having a positive bladder scope at my next appointment. There was no way that I was going to do chemotherapy and risk serious side effects. In addition to boosting my immune system through naturopathy, I was urgently searching for alternative cancer treatments. I discovered there are many different types of alternative therapy clinics in Mexico and Europe. A few examples of those advertised on the internet or in the media included:

- laetrile
- chelation
- Issels treatment
- nutritional therapy
- high-dose vitamins and dietary supplements
- metabolic therapy
- oxygen therapies
- hydrotherapy
- hyperthermia (high temperature therapy)

Many of the clinics offered a package of care that involved using a combination of treatments. Most of the programs are two to four weeks long and are like a luxury health spa. They were advertised as relaxing and caring. Although the clinic can't claim to cure your cancer, they promise that you will have individual care and that they can help you.

Often the package of care sounds attractive, but many of the reviewers stated that they could not maintain compliance with the very strict diet requirements. There were, however, reports of people with cancer leaving these clinics who were very happy with their care. Some even claimed that the treatment cured their cancer. I looked to the internet for these alternatives because I did not know anyone locally that could give me any professional guidance on alternative cures for cancer.

I just had such a great fear of the potential serious side effects of chemotherapy. I knew an individual fighting colon cancer who did three rounds of chemo. The cancer was cured, but she had to live 24/7 on oxygen because the chemo and radiation destroyed her lungs. I really felt that my fear was justified and was intent on proving that, with the power of the internet, I could find and follow a proven nutritional therapy protocol instead.

After days of research, I came across a program that looked promising to me. It was researched and developed by a well-known doctor from the United States who had practiced on the East Coast for 30 years before moving his practice to Mexico. It was insinuated that his restorative health practice was not approved by the FDA, and Mexico had an environment more conducive for his practice. He and his team had flourished there and had drawn many US citizens to his cancer-curing initiative.

My decision to engage with their institute was difficult. I really wanted to go to their facility in Mexico and do the full program, but I was not in a position to leave the country for four to six weeks while running my company. They offered a stay-at-home model of therapy I could follow that was a small portion of what they provided in Mexico. This way, I could remain home to work and be with my family. Since my wife and I owned a health and fitness company that provided nutritional supplements, it seemed logical that their nutritional plan could work for me and my cancer. I took the plunge and paid their fees to start the therapy.

In hindsight, it was a huge mistake for me to go to the internet. It was an overwhelming search; the internet was teeming with information on how to naturally cure yourself from cancer. You can find pretty much any opinion on any topic—just Google "does chocolate cure cancer" if you don't believe me. It also comes from pretty much any type of source: health organizations, merchants, private interest groups, government agencies, and even scam artists. Some are trying to inform.

Some are trying to make money. Some are even trying to deceive. The internet can be used for great good, and there were times it was a necessary and helpful tool in my health battles. But this time, unfortunately, I chose wrong. In my desperation, I chose the very thing that cancer loves.

The Protocol

Once I decide to do something, I do it 100%. This particular program required that and more. The protocol required daily juicing of fruits and vegetables. It had prescribed recipes that we were to follow. I was to consume thirteen juices a day. The grocery store shopping list was fascinating. Here's a list of organic produce that I needed for one week of juicing:

- Carrots 35–40 lbs
- Apples, 35–40 lbs
- Red cabbage, 1 head
- Green peppers, 8 medium
- Chard, 4 bunches
- Endive, 2 heads
- Grapefruit, 10–15 lbs
- Watercress, 2–3 bunches
- Oranges, 10–15 lbs
- Romaine, 7–14 heads

Oh, the looks we got as we wheeled our overloaded cart of produce through the checkout! They must've thought we were going to make salad for an army!

Each day required hours of work from both Carla and me to prepare it all. We'd get up early and start by soaking the produce in a plant-based, biodegradable formula. We'd cut and chop until our hands were sore, and it wasn't long until we had to start wearing gloves, as the citrus burned our raw, irritated skin.

We'd put it all into our juicing machine, discarding the pulp and filling 12 eight-ounce bottles, trying not to waste even one precious drop. By the end of our juicing production, our kitchen was a disaster. Every inch of counter space was used. It looked like a produce bomb had gone off in there. From start to finish, it took a total of four hours—two hours each—just to juice each day. It was a huge commitment that not only affected our demanding work schedules but also meant we had to give up our daily exercise routine, a true sacrifice for us both.

Drinking the juice was also a daunting task. I was required to drink 104 ounces of juice a day. Because of the sheer volume I was drinking, it was recommended I not drink any water. Two of the three juices did not taste good. Over time, I began to acquire a taste for them, but if I let any of the green juice sit for more than eight hours, it became bitter, and I had to force myself to chug it down. The key was not to smell it. Once I got a whiff, it was game over.

Within a month, we'd worn out both the juicing machine and any excitement we'd ever had for juicing. We bought another juicing machine and burned out that motor within a month. After some research, we purchased a commercial-grade juicer. We were in this for the long haul! We were completely convinced that juicing was the key to stopping the cancer growth. The age-old adage that "a little knowledge is a dangerous thing" definitely applied to us and our full-time commitment to my strict health protocols.

In addition to the juice, there was a long list of organic foods to buy each week. Organic was important, because studies showed that organic foods produce 20%–40% more antioxidants.[1] Basically, the program was plant-based and nutrient rich. I would be consuming 2,600 to 3,200 calories per day. Since I was going to follow the full therapeutic diet, it meant that I would be going through twenty pounds of food each day. Seventeen pounds of the raw foods would be made into juices, and three pounds would be turned into cooked foods. In essence, the goal was to have this diet high in potassium and low in sodium. A weekly shopping list for these foods would typically look like this.

- Leeks, 2 bunches
- Tomatoes, 10–15 lbs
- Onions, 20 per week
- Potatoes, 25 pounds
- Celery, 2–3 bunches
- Garlic, 4–6 or more bulbs
- Organic steel cut oats, 1 lb
- Raisins, 1 lb for 1 month
- Flaxseed oil
- Lemons
- Brown rice or quinoa
- Lentils

I was also allowed one banana per day and two slices of unsalted, non-fat, organic rye bread. Are you jealous yet?

---

1 "Organic Health Benefits Part 3: The Nutritional Benefits of Organic Fruits and Vegetables," The Organic Center, 12 October 2014, *https://www.organic-center.org/organic-health-benefits-part-3-the-nutritional-benefits-of-organic-fruits-and-vegetables/.*

I haven't even gotten to the list of prohibited foods, which included:

- Alcohol
- Berries
- Soy
- Avocados
- Sprouts
- Cucumbers
- Beans
- Candy and pastries (this one was really, really hard for me)
- Nuts and seeds
- Soda (including diet)
- Meat

Here's what a typical day's menu looked like.

Breakfast:

- Glass of orange juice or grapefruit juice
- Organic steel oats cooked in hot water, then let it sit until thickened. I could add a few raisins.
- Rye bread, plain

Lunch:

- Salad with a light dressing of flaxseed oil, lemon juice, and crushed garlic. (It took a while for me to acquire a taste for this.)
- 1–2 cooked vegetables (This was more complicated than you'd think. All the vegetables had to be cooked slowly over a low flame, without any added water. Cooking

this way preserves the natural flavor of the vegetables and keeps them easily digestible.)

- Baked potato (Don't get too excited. The only topping I was allowed was a cold salsa made from finely chopped tomato, green onions, cilantro, and lemon juice—another challenge that required some taste bud adaptation.)
- Soup
- Glass of juice

Dinner:

- (More of the same... It was lunch all over again.)
- Salad
- 1–2 cooked vegetables
- Baked potato
- Soup
- Glass of juice

Plus...ten more full jars of juice. The full protocol dictated exactly which juices to drink which hour of the day. It was intense! But I was willing. If it meant I didn't have to do chemo or radiation treatments, I'd guzzle all the thick, smelly veggie juice you could throw at me. Between the shopping, prepping, and eating/drinking, it felt like an additional full-time job. Carla did the shopping, and I helped with the prepping and cleanup, but in reality, Carla did the bulk of the work.

Carla

What did I get myself into? was the thought that repeated through my mind. I was already trying to balance a very full plate of responsibilities in my life, and now I was adding this crazy-demanding food prep. Honestly, it was like a full-time job. I was grateful that David helped for a couple hours in the morning with the juicing, but that was just the beginning of the work required to pull it off.

I've always loved cooking for my family and don't mind time spent in the kitchen, but this was a whole other level. If this had just been some diet protocol to help him lose weight, I could not have stuck it out. But in our minds, this was the treatment that was going to save his life. And I was willing to do whatever it took to do that.

David

Carla and I have always had a mutual understanding. She does the cooking and I do all the cleaning. If I cook, then we reverse the roles, and that has worked beautifully throughout our marriage. I learned how to cook as a teenager. My mom was a single parent and had to work full-time, and that left me to make dinner most days for our family. We were very poor, and we did not have a lot of ingredients.

One of my specialties was spaghetti. I boiled the noodles, added some hamburger, and topped it off with ketchup. I can laugh about this now, but back then, it got old night after night. Another favorite dish was tuna fish casserole. This involved mixing one can of tuna, a can of peas, and a can of mushroom soup together. Then I'd alternate layers of crushed potato chips and tuna mixture in a casserole dish and bake. To this day, I really struggle eating tuna fish. I was thankful for those cans from the local food pantry, but it wasn't always top-quality food.

Gratefully, my cooking repertoire has expanded, but Carla is the gourmet cook in our family. She loves cooking for our blended family of seven children and eighteen grandchildren. The first Sunday of every month, she prepares dinner and birthday desserts for the whole family. Carla is nothing short of amazing. I tried to be a good sport during all the months I followed this strict diet, but sitting with my bland baked potato and cold salsa while my family was dining on Carla's mouth-watering prime rib, fingerling potatoes dripping in hot butter and parsley, and homemade rolls was as close to torture as I hope I ever get.

I remained convinced that this diet would solve my cancer issue. We overlooked an important reality, however. It never occurred to us that sugar feeds cancer, and all that juice I was consuming was full of sugar. Juice is loaded with fructose, and although that's a naturally-occurring sugar, it still causes blood sugar to spike, especially when all the healthier parts of the fruit (such as the fiber in the pulp) get removed. I was drinking gallons of high-fructose liquid as I chugged down thirteen glasses of juice every day. I followed this daily menu with exactness. January... February... March... I ate the same foods day in and day out. All told, I followed the juicing and diet protocol every day for thirty months.

At first, all our efforts appeared to be working. We met with Dr. Oldroyd in April. This time, Carla wanted to be in the room to see and hear for herself how the exam went. We both agreed we'd never heard anything better than the words, "The bladder looks great, and there are no tumors."

The huge smile on Carla's face said it all. Once the equipment was out of me, Dr. Oldroyd left the room. Before I'd had a chance to clean up, with me still in my wet gown, Carla rushed over and gave me a huge hug. "We did it!" she cried. "It worked! David, NO TUMORS!" We relished this wonderful moment of victory. Over the past year, I'd had to endure two bladder surgeries and had a total of seventeen tumors removed. This clean scan made us think these days were behind us. The diet protocol was working! We went home to toast each other with a celebratory cup of juice.

CHAPTER 3

FRANKENSTEIN'S OFFICE

Before we'd left Dr. Oldroyd's office, he gave us some bad news. He was retiring. I smiled and congratulated him, but inside, my heart sank. When I asked him who I'd see moving forward and how often I needed to come in for a scope, he told me I'd be able to see his partner. He also said I'd need to continue coming every three months until I was tumor-free for a year.

From January to September, we complied 110% with the juicing and three-meals-a-day protocol. Choosing to stay at Dr. Oldroyd's practice became problematic. He retired at seventy years old. His partner of the same age was very experienced, and I tried to make an appointment with him, but no matter what I did, they pushed me to the doctor they'd hired to replace Dr. Oldroyd. This new doctor had just graduated from medical school with one year of residency under his belt. With tremendous anxiety, I finally relented and set an appointment for August 2016 with the new guy.

I arrived that day at the new urologist's office feeling dread and trepidation. The day was dry and hot, and I hesitated outside the office door. Was I sweating from the heat or from worry? Here I was, looking at my fifth bladder exam in eighteen months, but this time with a total stranger. It felt wrong, but wouldn't any new doctor I had to start over with be a crapshoot? If I'd had any clue how the next seven hours were going to unfold, I would have spent whatever time it took to find a different urologist. Unfortunately, I did not listen to my gut.

I was in a foul mood and didn't make any friendly small talk with anyone in the reception room. The young woman who took my co-pay could not have cared less about my plight. I took my receipt and found a seat. I hunkered down and looked out the windows facing the mountains.

The television in the room was set to a news program, and the reporters were droning on about all the negative happenings around the world. It added to my dark mood, and I slunk down even lower into the black vinyl padding of my stainless-steel chair. When I was called back to Dr. Oldroyd's old examination room, nostalgia set in as I looked around. I found myself really missing my good friend and doctor.

As I slowly undressed, I prayed for two things: First, that this new doctor would be competent. Second, that there would be no cancer in my bladder.

I assumed my position on the exam table. The new doctor sauntered in. His young, unwrinkled face, full head of dark brown hair, and 5'8" height (with shoes on) did nothing to bolster my confidence. It was like looking at a high school junior. He introduced himself to me, and I immediately started peppering him with questions. "Wow, how old are you? Is your best friend Doogie Houser?" I shouldn't have joked so inappropriately, but I couldn't help myself.

"Oh great, one of my very first patients turns out to be a Comedy Central guy, ha ha ha." He said "ha ha ha," in a deadpan, sarcastic monotone.

"You did graduate med school, right?" I asked, kidding, mostly. He assured me that, for the last year, he'd been finishing his residency with an oncologist. But he'd just admitted I was one of his first patients, so that did little to ease my concerns.

Once again, I was being manhandled, and I did not like it. It reminded me of all those times in high school, having to stand naked in the showers with all of the other boys going through puberty. It was so embarrassing then, and it was embarrassing now. I just sucked it up and stared at the ceiling, concentrating on the rectangular ceiling tiles. This doctor wasn't nearly as gentle as he awkwardly maneuvered the equipment up into my bladder.

My last appointment with Dr. Oldroyd had been so easy—in and out in no time. This time it all seemed to be taking forever. I was staring at those fascinating ceiling tiles and avoiding looking at the toddler-doctor's face. He was in there for several minutes when I heard him say, "I see a good-sized tumor."

With my eyes still focused on the ceiling, I said, "Are you kidding me?" I tried to keep my voice calm, but I was immediately super angry. I wasn't angry with this new doctor (yet), but the betrayal I felt at hearing those words after my complete dedication to such a stringent healthy eating protocol for the last seven months was acute. I had come today totally expecting to be clean of any cancerous tumors in my bladder. His calm pronouncement whiplashed through me and knocked me totally off-center.

That was just the beginning of the seven-hour nightmare. First, this new doctor decided to do something that Dr. Oldroyd never did. After pulling out the equipment from my body, he said, "I need to get a biopsy before I do surgery." I honestly had no idea what to say to that comment. The only words that came out of my mouth were, "How and when do you do that?" His reply was, "Right now."

If I'd had any clue what was going to happen over the next seven hours, I would've shoved that doctor away from me, thrown on my clothes, and ran out of that building to never return again. If someone had told me all that I was about to endure, I wouldn't have believed them.

I'll leave it to your imagination to decide how you get a biopsy with a tiny pair of scissors and a scope. Naively, I let an unskilled doctor perform an internal biopsy on me just minutes after an already painful procedure. It was like watching a kid playing an arcade game—he'd wince with each snip as if he'd missed a shot fired at some pixelated alien. What was happening inside my bladder was straight out of Dante's Inferno. We were literally in the Seventh Circle of hell: "Violence." It took him nine tries before he got his tissue sample. Nine...

Finally, with a sigh of relief, the doctor blurted out, "I got it!" and they started to remove the equipment. The doctor proudly held up the small tissue sample that hung from the end of the flexible grips as if to say, "Ta-da! Presenting... your biopsy!"

He put the tissue in a small sample bottle filled with fluid and said, "We will get this sample right off to verify that it is cancer." I blinked, still focused on the large amount of blood accumulating on the table. He continued, "I am pretty confident that it is cancer based on your history." *No kidding... You think?* I wanted to shake him and say, "You forced me to go through this whole embarrassing and painful mess for nothing?!"

In the bathroom, the blood loss continued. I stared at myself in the mirror, taking in my shaved bald head, the dark bags under my eyes, the scar on my right jawline from a previous squamous cancer procedure, and my pale complexion from the horror of the past hour. Ominous thoughts raced through my mind. I had cancer again. I had cancer. Again. As if that weren't bad enough, this doctor just butchered a simple procedure. What I'd just endured was indescribably painful. It felt like all the stars in the universe had aligned against me.

Driving home, I called Carla and told her the whole ugly story. The unfortunate series of events really shook her up. She was as shocked as I was that the cancer had returned, and I was facing another surgery. She tried to make sense of his decision to do the biopsy; perhaps it was because he only did surgeries on Tuesdays, so there was time to get a biopsy result? She felt very bad for me, which made me feel a little better, and we both hoped the bleeding would stop soon.

We had no such luck. For the next several hours, my pain did not subside, and the intense bleeding continued. I called the office and told the nurse, "I think I'm bleeding out." She asked if I could be at the office at 4:30.

While Carla and I were driving back to the urologist's office, we discussed how frustrating it was to be looking at a third surgery. "Let's not tell anybody about this!" I insisted. I was just so sick and tired of talking about my bladder cancer. The conversations just go on and on. Nobody ever seems to want to talk about anything else.

Because of our business, we get invited to a lot of lunch and dinner events. People watch what I eat and don't eat, what I drink and don't drink. And I knew everyone would question why all the hard work of the juicing and diet wasn't working. It truly gets exhausting. At this point, I was over it—all of it.

Carla

I did cry. It's interesting: With the first cancer diagnosis, I had some tears, but not much. I was able to remain pretty positive and optimistic. This time felt totally different. This one felt like all the doom and gloom talk you hear from people, that you never get rid of bladder cancer, you have to deal with it the rest of your life, blah, blah, blah. It felt heavy.

I didn't want to call my family and friends again and tell them the cancer was back. I didn't want to ask everyone to pray for us—yet again. We'd already asked for so many prayers between the other two big surgeries David had had in the past twelve months. I just couldn't do it again. We decided not to say anything to anyone.

I'd always thought it was strange when I found out someone had a major health problem after the fact—like someone whose dad had cancer, but they didn't know until he died—but now I kind of got it. Once you have cancer, it's all anyone wants to talk about. It's all-consuming. Everyone tells you their cancer stories about their mom, their cousin, their friend, and everyone has opinions on what you should do and not do, which books you need to read. It's exhausting. Once I said to a well-meaning friend, "You know, I have twelve grandkids. I'd love to talk about them! Anything, really, besides cancer!"

We decided to only tell our family and a few close friends. I was very nervous this time. Why did he keep going from zero tumors to one or more every few months? My other concern was the anesthesia. David simply didn't handle it well. Each surgery seemed harder for him to come out of it. It also had a dramatic effect on his short-term memory. Our family and even some employees had noticed this after the last time. Even to my stalwartly optimistic self, more tumors seemed like a devastating blow.

David

We walked into the office arm in arm. Carla decided to wait in the reception room while the same nurse from that morning led me back. Instead of heading to the exam room I'd been in multiple times before, however, we turned right. Before I knew it, I was walking into Dr. Frankenstein's experimental chamber.

I'm not kidding. Had the lights been dimmed and scary music playing, it would've been a scene straight out of a horror movie. To my left stood an exam table with a raised back and two massive, arm-like appendages attached to either side. A big white bucket hung from the ceiling by an orange bungee cord, with a huge piece of equipment of some sort on the other side. Two lone black chairs adorned the wall beyond the table, and there was one small, opaque window. The walls were bare. I gaped at what was very obviously a makeshift procedure room. The nurse told me to undress and put on a blue gown that tied in the back, then left to get the doctor.

It felt surreal. My head was spinning with the craziness of it all—possibly compounded by the loss of blood at this point. The doctor and nurse came in, and in my mind I was screaming, *Not again!* I was even more aggravated that a female nurse had to be part of whatever was going to happen to me in that room. I was in this nightmare because the doctor messed up!

I was told to sit on the table between the two appendages. Before I could make any conversation, the doctor said, "I've got to go back into the bladder and cauterize the area to stop your bleeding." My mind did not fully register what this meant.

"Is this my only option?" I asked in dismay.

Dr. Newbie was stoic. "Yep. Only way to stop the bleeding. Now lean back and put your legs up here." He pointed to the cold and uncomfortable contraptions on either side of me. At this point, you should be extra grateful to my editor, who made me remove the brutal details that followed. I'll just say that cauterization within an internal organ requires a lot of electricity and a flame.

Sweating and trying not to hyperventilate, I wondered why I wasn't given a sedative. Later, I found out I should have been given a sedative for that morning's biopsy and both a sedative and an antibiotic for the cauterization, especially since I typically get a severe bladder infection after a bladder exam. I received nothing of the sort from Dr. Frankenstein.

An hour of painful and unsuccessful internal camera positioning was followed by six missed attempts, and I smelled something burning. With a start, I realized the thing burning was me! He was barbecuing my bladder! I glanced at him. He was looking at the monitor with a look of dissatisfaction. The two reluctant nurses looked completely bewildered.

Finally, on the seventh try, the doctor said, "Well, I think I was finally able to cauterize it." He looked at me. "You're not on any blood thinners, are you?" *Uh, isn't it a little too late to be asking that question, moron?* I saw the nurses worriedly glance at each other. Thankfully, I was not.

The nurses looked relieved, and then they gave me that look, like, "You poor soul." All I could do was mouth "thank you" to them. I completely ignored Dr. Frankenstein. There was no way I would ever step foot in that facility again as long as I live on this earth. Once he pulled the lever and released the stirrups, my legs and groin sagged together in relief.

I was in shock as I got dressed. Pulling on my socks, I noticed the time on my watch—6:15 p.m. I realized I'd just endured seven hours of humiliation and pain. As I slid on my shoes and shirt, I registered how much pain I was truly enduring. Not waiting for the doctor or nurses, I shuffled out to the empty waiting room. Carla could tell I was very upset.

Without any explanation, I looked at her and said, "We need to leave. Right now."

"What? What happened? Are you okay?"

"Just get me out of here."

She picked up her purse and followed as I limped to the elevator. "How much pain are you in? And what's that smell?" She sniffed the air. "David, you smell like burning flesh!" Honestly, I was inches from losing it. Having Carla there was the only thing keeping me from going berserk. I kept saying to myself, *Don't stain the Meine name. Don't stain the Meine name*, the mantra my mom had taught me years ago as a child.

Once we were safely inside the closed elevator, I began recounting the horrible tale of my Frankenstein nightmare. I asked her to drive since I was in so much pain, and I continued the story all the way home. As we pulled into the garage, I asked her to get me my pain medication and headed straight to our bedroom. She brought me two Lortabs and some sleeping medicine. I gulped it down, curled up in the fetal position, and prayed for the pain to subside.

My body was hammered. In less than twenty months, I'd had back surgery, two cancer surgeries, multiple painful cystoscopies (including Frankenstein's butchery), and now a third cancer surgery looming ahead of me. Carla was an absolute saint through it all. Being my caretaker couldn't have been easy.

Typically, I'm a very positive person, and I love people. But through these health challenges, I'm sure there were many days when I was grumpy from the pain. I'd also had real struggles with short-term memory loss from all the anesthesia I'd undergone. This didn't just affect me—it affected our family members, friends, and our business. I was often in the limelight as the Founder and CEO, and during this time, an international company was making bids to buy us out. It was a lot to handle.

My faith in modern medicine was shaken. I knew I required medical help if I wanted to live, but I felt more hesitation than ever about entrusting my health—my life, my ability to have a future—to just any medical professional. All of this just confirmed my decision about not doing chemotherapy. I was more adamant about that than ever. There just had to be another way.

CHAPTER 4

A LITTLE HOPE IS A POWERFUL THING

I spiraled over the next few months. My mind cycled through a constant reel of bleak and futile thoughts: Why me? Why am I in this predicament, fighting something that I cannot see? Why is this cancer coming back, and why can't I even find a competent doctor? Why isn't the cancer-fighting diet working? It felt like I was drowning in an overwhelming, unsolvable dilemma.

A few days after the Frankenstein experience, I was back at the pharmacy to pick up my prescription for the inevitable bladder infection I always got after a procedure. As the pharmacist handed me the little white bag, I thought about the many times I'd been handed a similar white bag over the years. So often, a doctor had instantly prescribed something to treat one of my health problems. Surely there was a better, preventative way?

I'd tried talking to doctors over the years about alternative, preventative methods, but nobody ever wanted to engage in the conversation. Whenever I'd asked a doctor about a dietary solution, a natural solution versus a prescribed fix, I'd get a blank stare. Most doctors I know seem to think their job is to diagnose and then provide a prescription drug that will solve the problem or provide a pain drug until the symptoms go away. Even if you ask about potential nutraceuticals, they typically say they are a waste of money. I had one doctor state that the only thing supplements do is make your pee more colorful.

As I gulped down the large, white pill I'd been prescribed today, I began to seriously question the diet I'd been on for seven months. *Just give it more time,* I told myself. *It's going to eventually work.* My thinking was the epitome of blind faith.

Despite the cancer, life remained very busy. I continued to train for my upcoming competitive cycling events, unwilling to give up what had become a lifeline for me. During this time, Carla and I also negotiated the sale of our business. Whatever spare time I had left was spent intensely Googling CANCER SOLUTIONS. The internet seemed to be my last hope for solving my overwhelming dilemma.

One day, I noticed a sponsored link that advertised a chain of hospitals specializing in cancer. They had multiple locations across the US, and one of their locations was in Phoenix, Arizona. They claimed to have a multidisciplinary approach, including new immunotherapy treatments and genomic testing.

After several hours of reading the content on their web pages and watching testimonial videos, I felt confident enough to click the link to schedule a consultation. There was an opening the following day, and I felt an instant sense of relief just knowing I had the appointment. I told Carla, and she came over and wrapped her arms around me. After a long hug, she pulled back and gave me a relieved look. We were both desperate for some good news.

That night was the first time since enduring Dr. Frankenstein that I got a decent night's sleep. I awoke the next morning with a sense of optimism. That first phone call with the cancer clinic went well, and my optimism remained. We set an appointment for another phone call with one of their doctors for the following week, which also went well and bolstered my confidence in this clinic. After that call, they scheduled a follow-up call with their "Becoming-a-Patient Specialist."

After the very friendly representative explained the process, I felt exhausted and overwhelmed. Nothing related to cancer was easy! However, they had an opening for surgery in three weeks. Having been to Phoenix in my twenties, I had experienced first-hand how extremely hot August can be. But I didn't care. I was feeling a bit of hope about my cancer, and a little hope can be a powerful thing. I gave her my insurance information and hung up, convinced we had found a great solution.

When you have a potentially life-threatening illness, you'd think that the sickness itself would be the hardest thing to deal with. You'd think that the physical battles would be the worst challenge you'd face. Sometimes that's true. However, the emotional trauma and fatigue that comes from having to battle insurance companies regarding authorizations and declined procedures and loopholes just suck the life out of you. It makes any physical battle you may be facing infinitely worse. Several days later, I got a call from the hospital, and this time their representative was all business. "Do you have a secondary health insurance policy?" she asked.

My primary insurance wouldn't approve that particular hospital facility for the surgery. My heart completely sank. I'd been mentally preparing myself for the surgery and was anxious to have it done. Perhaps I could afford to pay out of pocket. "Do you have a financing plan? How much does the surgery cost?" I asked. They'd have to get back to me about the full cost of the outpatient program—more uncertainty and more waiting.

I felt that sick, anxious feeling in the pit of my stomach return. After talking to Carla, I realized the costs involved would include much more than just the surgery. We would have to be there two days early for tests. We'd need a hotel, rental car, airfare, and food for at least four days. And that was the best-case scenario. If anything went wrong, the cost could be significantly higher.

I started spiraling, and the negative thoughts that I'd been battling returned. *What am I getting myself into?* I thought. I was also feeling incredibly impatient, and waiting days for information was getting old. You'd think that with everything I'd been through over the past twenty months, I could deal with the unexpected and unknown. I had gotten good at acting calm on the outside, but inside, I was slipping into a hole of depression.

By the time they called me back, I had researched all the costs of the trip to Phoenix and thought I was ready for their numbers. The rep calmly informed me, "The best estimate we can give you is $55,000 if there are no complications. You'll need to decide fairly soon. We won't be able to hold your spot for surgery much longer." When I heard that, I almost tipped backward out of my chair. I was beyond agitated—not at her but at the whole situation. To remain polite, I needed to get off the phone as quickly as possible.

Carla assured me we would figure it out, but this blow knocked me over. I'd lost all motivation to work with the hospital. It was as if someone had let all the air out of a balloon. I felt empty and deflated.

That night we went to a surprise birthday party with some friends at a restaurant in Provo. One couple, Walt and Carole, were from out of town. We didn't know them very well, and we were surprised when we heard they were coming. Walt had been diagnosed with stage 4 prostate cancer, and the last time we'd seen him, he looked terrible. We couldn't imagine that he would be up for a dinner party. They arrived late, and we were completely stunned when he walked in. He looked like a totally different man than the one we'd seen a few months before. We all stood to give Walt and Carole big hugs.

"Whoa!" I said, "You look amazing!"

"I feel amazing!" he responded vigorously.

After dinner, we lingered at the table, everyone animatedly chatting. Carla and I were seated near Walt, and I commented again about how great he looked. He shared some of his cancer journey of the past two years with us.

"I found a new doctor," he confided. "He's given me eight more years to live, and he's confident that during those eight years, there will be additional things we can do to extend my life."

I felt a nudge deep inside. Could it be possible? The last time we'd seen him, we'd thought he was close to death. Instead, he looked happy and full of renewed life. Everyone was talking over each other, but I wanted to hear every word Walt said. I also wanted to ask him to tell me more.

Before I could ask, Walt leaned closer to me. "David, how is your battle with bladder cancer going?"

Knowing the restaurant was probably getting anxious to have our table, I gave him a short, five-minute version. As I was winding up, I asked him, "So who is this new doctor that you found?"

Walt shared that, through a long series of events, he'd been referred to Dr. Jay Bishoff in Salt Lake City. "If it weren't for him, I'd be dead," Walt declared. We were quiet for a moment, digesting this very sobering thought. Then he offered, "Would you like Dr. Bishoff's contact information?"

"Yes!" I responded immediately. Knowing the urgency of my situation, Walt said I could use his name to get in, as the doctor was very busy. He also explained that this doctor had specialized equipment that no other doctor in the state of Utah had. A spark of hope once again started to glimmer inside of me, fueled by this new possibility. Could this be the miracle I needed? "Thank you," I said as Carla and I hugged him and his wife. "And I'm so grateful things are looking up for you."

I called Dr. Bishoff's office first thing the next day. The receptionist was very frustrating. No matter what I said, she insisted the doctor was not accepting any new patients. She kept trying to move me to another doctor. I tried everything, including dropping Walt's name. Exasperated, she finally said she would transfer me to the head nurse.

When Greta, the nurse, came on the phone, I pleaded my case as if my life were on the line. Because it was, and I was not going to take no for an answer. I'd done my research early that morning and knew his practice took our health insurance. After five minutes of conversation—which was pretty much me talking and her listening—she said she'd get the scheduler and see if there were any openings for new patients. I hadn't realized I'd been holding my breath until she put me on hold. Exhaling, I started praying they'd somehow get me in.

After a few minutes, they both came on the line. The scheduler asked how soon I needed an appointment. I explained that my previous urologist had retired, that a new cancer tumor had been found in my bladder, and I needed surgery. My heart was pounding, and I had my next argument ready as they looked through the dates. "Mr. Meine, how would October 4th at 10:00 am work for you?" I paused. That was three weeks away and the first day of my cycling events at the Utah Huntsman Senior Games, where I was slated to compete, but this was way more important.

"I will take it!" I exclaimed. I thanked them profusely, hung up, and called Carla. As soon as she answered the phone, I said, "We got our miracle! I have an opportunity to meet with Dr. Bishoff on October 4th!"

"Oh, honey!" she gasped. "That is so wonderful! And such a relief!"

Now I just had to exercise some more patience and wait for the first of many meetings with Dr. Jay Bishoff, an Oncologist Urologist. I was hopeful—hopeful that this doctor could remove the cancer through surgery and hopeful that he would help us figure out why the cancer kept coming back. That hope got me through.

CHAPTER 5

A SIDESTEP INTO FOOT PROBLEMS

Please indulge me in a little side trip back to 1999 regarding another serious health problem that began fifteen years prior to my battle with cancer. I had no reason to believe the two were connected, and it would be many years before I'd be able to put it all together. However, I have since learned that all my health issues are closely intertwined. They are each an important thread in the overall tapestry of my health.

Each symptom was a thread in a common but devious underlying cause. And that cause was addiction.

It's not the sort of addiction you might be thinking. As someone with a strong genetic history of alcoholic ancestors, I'd always considered myself lucky that I've never struggled with addiction. Drugs and alcohol have never tempted me. But I was an addict nonetheless. One of the most important turning points of my life was eventually coming to learn that within the interconnectedness of my health issues loomed two gargantuan addictions. These addictions would become my greatest battles in life.

The story below was an important stepping stone in my journey to overcoming this battle.

Winter, 1999

I looked at my watch. It was only 3:30 p.m. How was I going to survive the rest of this meeting? My feet were killing me. It felt like someone was holding a blow torch against the bottom of them. I had no idea why or what was causing the intense pain. I clenched my jaw and tried to focus, but it was completely distracting me from the meeting.

I slowly lifted my left foot and used my toes to surreptitiously push the shoe off my other foot. I crossed my right ankle over my knee, again moving slowly so that no one would notice, and rubbed my foot through my sock. My client's IT Director was droning on about their current data center solutions, and everyone around me was listening intently.

I snuck a peek at my foot to see if there was anything visually that could be causing the burning sensation, but there didn't appear to be any needles or other small pieces of weaponry attached to my sock. I rubbed my hand back and forth underneath my toes and along the arch. It didn't feel hot to the touch, even though my feet were both on fire. I quietly slipped off my other shoe, which diminished the pain to a point where I could at least attempt to refocus on the meeting.

This ridiculous problem with my feet had been going on for some time now. Not only did my feet hurt every day like clockwork in the late afternoon, but they were also unbearable at night. The slightest touch of a blanket or sheets hurt tremendously, and I would carefully roll up the bedding to try and find some relief. I'd gotten a referral for an appointment with a neurologist, but not until January, and it couldn't come soon enough.

I knew of no one else with this strange condition with whom to compare notes. I took lots of Advil, and my doctor prescribed Naproxen (another form of Ibuprofen) for the pain. I was typically consuming three doses of 800 mgs each per day. These over-the-counter and prescription pain meds would take the pain level from a ten down to a six, making it at least bearable.

I'd started to train for triathlons the previous summer (no matter how much pain I was in, I couldn't stand the thought of giving up my training), and at my first race I'd won a really awesome indoor treadmill. I kept wondering if running on it had somehow caused this serious foot condition. I was anxious to ask the neurologist.

When the day of my appointment finally arrived, I assessed the doctor I'd been referred to as he entered the room. I was wary, as he was young and new to the practice, but all the other neurologists in my area were either booked out for months or not accepting new patients. This guy was obviously a man of few words, and he quietly reviewed the paperwork I'd filled out.

He glanced at me. "Are your feet hurting right now?" he asked.

"On a pain scale of one to ten, they're at about a four," I responded. "I took off my shoes while waiting for you. I take off my shoes a lot. It helps the pain a little."

He offered no response, reaching into his white medical jacket and pulling out a small instrument. He hit below my kneecap with the triangular rubber mallet. My leg jerked in response. He did the same to the other leg, the small kick seeming to be what he was looking for.

He did a series of tests using a tuning fork and then gauged my ability to balance, all the while remaining silent. Finally, he said, "I am going to recommend a prescription for pain, diabetes testing, and order an electromyography." After so much silence, it now seemed he was saying everything all at once. I grappled with what question to ask first.

"What is that big-long-word procedure that I need?"

He quietly chuckled and said with a smile, "You can just call it an EMG." When he saw that still wasn't registering for me, he elaborated. I tried to follow all of his explanations about the tests and the bloodwork, and the meds. "You should see a decrease in the foot pain you're experiencing. Let's get back together as soon as you can schedule the EMG, and also go over the diabetes results and see how you're doing on the medicine." I gave him a weak smile. I felt like I'd been run over by a horse.

I made an appointment for the EMG on my way out. As I was opening the door to my car, it dawned on me that I had no idea what relevance a diabetes blood test had on my feet. I slid into the seat and secured my seatbelt while more questions pelted my mind. How does it work? Is it painful? Are there any side effects of the medication? I was feeling like an idiot for not having asked more questions, but there's just too much to comprehend when you only get a few minutes with the doctor. Oh well. I figured I'd just have to wait until my next appointment with him in two weeks.

I arrived for my EMG appointment two weeks later. I was fairly nervous, especially since I'd had a bad reaction to the medication he'd prescribed me. I only took it for three days, and it did nothing for the pain while making me feel all-around yucky and miserable.

The doctor entered, pushing a rolling cart. I flashed back to a black-and-white episode of Flash Gordon from my childhood. It looked like a freak robot, with wires and coils sticking out of it on all sides, ready to torture me.

"How are you doing?" he greeted me.

"Not great. I had a bad reaction to the medicine."

He remained completely unfazed. "Sometimes that happens," he said nonchalantly. "I have another medicine that should work." He tapped his cheek with his forefinger. "How bad has the pain been in the last two weeks?"

"It's the same," I responded. "It's really bad, and it's distracting me at work. People are noticing. They're starting to ask about why I constantly take off my shoes." He remained silent, so I marched ahead with my monologue. "The medicine didn't seem to make any difference as far as the pain goes. But it made me feel super crappy." I continued to describe the side effects while he pulled out the tuning fork and repeated the same tests he'd done before.

I finished my rant of information and stared at the ominous computer cart while he made some notes. Finally, he flipped my chart closed and said, "Okay, let's do the EMG." That was when I noticed the long needle on the end of a wire. What had I gotten myself into? Why hadn't I done any research about the EMG?

"So, how does this whole thing," I paused and nodded my head toward the freaky contraption, "work? And, how long does this take?" Even as I said it, I realized I was asking way too little, way too late.

"The entire procedure should take between thirty and sixty minutes." He went into professor mode, his voice an emotionless monotone. "There are two components to an EMG test: the nerve conduction study and the needle electrodes EMG." Those words set off a red flag in my brain. Needle electrodes? That sounded like part of a mad scientist's torture chamber. He was still talking, and I hurried to catch up with what he was saying. He provided a long explanation of it all, but all I could do was focus on how many times he said the word "needles." My whole body was on high alert.

He did the electrode testing first, which wasn't too bad. I was just starting to relax a little when he said, "I'm going to start at the middle of your thigh and stick this needle through the skin into the muscle."

At that, my heart rate went into overdrive. "Are you serious?!" I asked, incredulous. It was more of an accusation than a question as I stared at him. He did, indeed, look dead serious. I tried again. "Are you just going to stick me in this one place?"

"No, I will be going about four inches at a time all the way down to your feet." I'm sure it was impossible for him to miss the look of pure terror on my face. "The good news is that it's going to hurt you a lot more than me," he deadpanned.

Needless to say, I didn't find it funny. "So you're basically saying I'm going to experience multiple, painful bee stings all the way down to my feet?"

"Yup," he said, completely nonplussed. I was trying to take deep, calming breaths without them noticing. If I'd had any idea what I was getting myself into, I would have chickened out for sure. There was no way out now, so I just had to suck it up and try to grin and bear it. I felt like I'd just become a live version of a voodoo doll.

By the time the test was done, my gown was soaked through with sweat. It was even more excruciating than I'd imagined. If I hadn't still felt the pain from the multiple needle sticks, I would have thought I needed to wake up from a really terrible nightmare.

Once I was dressed, the doctor returned and invited me to sit in one of the two chairs in the room. He pulled the other one over so we could face each other. He looked down, apparently trying to collect his thoughts. Before he could pull it together, I interjected, "That is a pretty brutal testing procedure. Was it worth it?"

"Well, I would not want to go through it." Again, the compassion was astounding from this guy. I then noticed a file in his hands. He pulled out a paper and said, "This is the lab report for your diabetes test. It came back negative."

Patience has never been my greatest virtue, and this guy had already tested mine to its limits. Without waiting for him to explain further, I asked, "What does diabetes have to do with my foot pain?"

"What we're doing is ruling out possibilities. We now know you don't have a condition called diabetic peripheral neuropathy." Dr. Quiet had finally found all his words, and he dove into a lengthy explanation about a condition that I didn't have.

I was getting very antsy. When he paused his dissertation, I jumped in with, "Okay, so what *do* I have?"

He took a deep breath. "Since we have ruled out DPN, that leaves us with peripheral neuropathy, which means that you have nerve damage in your feet that can be from genetics or some traumatic injury."

I grimaced and then worked to unclench my jaw. "Is there a treatment for this peripheral neuropathy?"

He shook his head. "I'm sorry to say that there is not a quick fix."

He didn't say anything else. Was he waiting for me to respond? I looked at him dumbly and muttered, "I cannot believe this is happening to me."

He responded flatly, "I'm going to give you a prescription for Lyrica. It should help with the pain."

Great. Another medication. "I hate medicine," I said. "Can you tell me what the side effects of this one are?"

"Dizziness, drowsiness, unsteadiness, memory loss, lack of coordination, difficulty speaking, viral infections, tremors... to list a few."

I began to nervously chuckle and shake my head back and forth, my trademark response when presented with a conundrum. "Do you have any other questions?" he asked.

"Aahhhhh, I don't know at the moment." I was already reeling from information overload.

"I'll need to see you every six months to see if the peripheral neuropathy progresses any further up your feet and how the medicine is working."

That was it? That was all he had? "Okay," I said shakily. He stood up, indicating the appointment was over. I left his office with a new diagnosis, very little understanding, and yet another prescription.

It has been two decades since my original peripheral neuropathy diagnosis. The doctor who diagnosed me was a specialist in the study of nerves and muscles. But the concept that the food we eat and beverages we drink affect our nerves and muscles seemed to make no difference to him or to most of the medical professionals I've worked with since. No questions about diet or lifestyle were ever asked. He was unfazed by the amount of over-the-counter pain medication, or NSAIDs, I was consuming each day.

Over the past twenty years, I have seen various neurologists. Not one ever broached the subject of diet or offered any suggestions as to how to get me off toxic medications such as Lyrica and other pain relievers. And they definitely never made the connection between my intense pain and the addictions that fed them. It was years before I learned that my daily consumption of multiple NSAIDs, along with my intense daily cravings for sugar, were major addictions that were actually feeding my pain and exacerbating my health issues.

Since this diagnosis, I've had multiple additional health problems. I didn't realize it then, but these health issues weren't isolated incidents. They were interconnected by common threads, which, once understood and armed with the correct knowledge, allowed me to break the dangerous cycle I was in, overcome my addictions, and get a handle on my health. Overcoming these addictions (which we'll discuss in more detail in upcoming chapters) is one of the hardest things I've ever done, but it probably saved my life. Without question, it has increased the quality of my life. I've even been able to mitigate 95% of my foot pain—without medication.

Have you had various, seemingly unrelated health challenges in your life? Do you see your primary care physician for in-and-out appointments and always leave well-supplied with a new set of prescriptions? Have you learned to live with certain amounts of discomfort, even pain, because there is no "quick fix" or cure? I've been there. I spent years there. And I am so thoroughly grateful to be on the other side.

CHAPTER 6

ADHD: MY SUPERPOWER

Please allow me another purposeful flashback that is part of the overall tapestry of my health. Once again, a seemingly unrelated issue I'd had years before played an important role in my holistic picture of wellness.

Have you ever had one of those years where you wish you could have a do-over? 1999 would certainly qualify as one of those years for me. On top of my struggle with severe pain in my feet and the difficult neuropathy diagnosis, it was time to address some additional demons.

It had been five years since my divorce, and it hadn't been pretty. During the last two years of my marriage, we had worked with a counselor. After the divorce, I continued to work with that counselor on my own. She'd helped me identify some unresolved issues from my childhood. Because of the deep emotional scars I had from being abandoned as a teen, I found myself repeatedly being attracted to the wrong type of person. Or not feeling worthy of the right kind. I was impulsive in my relationships, making big decisions on a whim that left hearts broken, including mine. On top of this, I was a single "Disneyland dad" and only got my four children every other weekend and one night a week. I didn't feel like I was doing any of it well.

I had the same pattern in business. Impulsiveness can sometimes be useful in a business situation. I was super high-energy and a big-idea guy. In some ways, it's like being a gambler. There are times you win big. But if you're on a losing streak and can't stop, it can create serious problems. And, when something didn't go well, I'd jump ship. Being a serial entrepreneur had some frustrating consequences for my employees and me.

The best thing I ever did was to admit I needed help. Before seeking therapy, I had tried so hard to do it on my own and could not figure out why I couldn't change my behavior. Eventually, I turned to the professionals and found a competent psychologist and psychiatrist. Long story short, my psychiatrist, Cathy, diagnosed me with ADHD (Attention Deficit-Hyperactivity Disorder). When she delivered the news, you could've knocked me over with a feather. "Are you serious, Cathy? That diagnosis has a very negative connotation. It's not even socially acceptable!"

Cathy gave me a tolerant smile and brushed some stray strands of blonde hair out of her eyes. Looking up and to the right, not meeting my eyes, she said, "David, we can manage this with medication. Nobody will need to know anything about this diagnosis."

At this point, you've probably already figured out that I don't have a super great filter. I might sometimes—okay, maybe oftentimes—speak before I think. What happened next is a great example of this. "Why in the world do I have to medicate for ADHD? It's not like I'm some hyperactive child!"

She scrunched up her eyebrows and looked like a parent patiently disciplining a little boy. "David, do you want to improve your behavior? You came to us of your own volition to get help."

Chastened, I tried to keep my emotions in check. I slowly nodded that I would follow her advice but had to clamp my jaw shut to keep from saying anything else inappropriate.

"Okay, David, we're going to put you on a proven drug for ADHD called Ritalin."

"I've heard of that, but only as a medication for children." I looked past her at the three framed degrees on her wall, trying to remind myself of her credibility. But all I could think about were the many bad things I'd heard about that particular medication. In the 1990s, it had become a popular go-to drug but now had a pretty negative reputation, as far as I knew. I knew parents whose children had had very negative experiences with it. How could I politely but firmly decline the prescription?

Instead, I simply asked, "What are the side effects?"

Without hesitation, she launched into the list. "There are a few: nervousness, agitation, anxiety, insomnia, stomach pain, loss of appetite... some people lose weight."

Wow, such wonderful things to look forward to. Cathy could tell I had lost focus and was less than pleased. She handed me a handwritten prescription. I took it and crumpled it in my pocket. "David," she said quietly, again in her mom voice. "This will be a great step for you to take to get the results you're looking for."

I managed to contain my anger, which had been building throughout the appointment until I left the office. I got in my car and slammed the door. *I am one of* those *people,* I thought. Did I require medication to control my behavior? How had this happened? I felt completely disgusted with myself. Why was the universe against me? Instead of going back to work, I went home to brood.

I laid on my bed in the dark for several hours, unable to sleep. I finally gave up and got on my computer to research more about this ADHD diagnosis. I sat there with the cursor blinking in the search bar for a few minutes, then finally typed, "Attitudes about ADHD diagnosis?" I was pretty hung up on the perception of those diagnosed with what I thought was such a negative disorder.

Google confirmed my fears, and I was appalled by the search results. I read article after article, all filled with negativity. I read words like "severely impulsive," "restless and inattentive behavior," "aggressive," and "disturbed." There were even words like "monsters" and "zombies," referring to those treated with prescription medications. But the number-one word I noticed from reading hundreds of articles was "shame." My own shame grew as I read.

I was especially disturbed when I read about a survey where most participants considered ADHD to be a mental illness. Was I mentally ill? That thought crossed a line for me, and it shamed me into filling the prescription Cathy had given me.

I had it filled on a Thursday and took the first pill that night. I took a second pill on Friday morning and went to work. At about one in the afternoon, I couldn't take it any longer and had to leave. For some reason, there was a beehive in my lower legs. There is no other way to describe it. I went home, and in frustration, I jumped on my bike and rode as hard and as fast as I could for ten miles, trying to get the horrible sensation to subside in my legs. The last three miles, I did a full-out sprint, but the cycling did nothing to relieve the incessant buzzing and whirring of those bees.

I'd had a building sense of anxiety all day. By that evening, I could no longer stand it. The only thing I could think to do at that point was to call Cathy. It was Friday night, and I called her office. No one answered, so I stayed on long enough to hear the recording with the number to call in an emergency. I dialed the number, but all I could do was leave a message.

Several hours later, Cathy called me back, and I described what I was going through. "You're having an adverse reaction to the medication," she said. *No, duh,* I thought sarcastically. "I'm sorry you're going through this, but it takes trial and error to get you on the right medication."

I immediately responded, "Oh, no! I am done with taking medication for my mental illness."

That got her attention. "David, I don't know where you got that idea. That is so far from the truth! This is not nearly as negative as you're thinking. Please, just throw the rest of the medication out, and relax for the rest of the weekend. I'll have someone call and schedule you to come in next week. We'll sort this out."

As politely as possible, I managed, "I look forward to it," and hung up. It wasn't until Sunday that I started feeling normal again. It's hard to believe how down I got on myself. It was like a switch had been kicked on by a tempest of negativity.

Some good did come out of it, though, as I started putting some things from my past together. I remembered how I seemed to constantly be in trouble during my early elementary years. I became well acquainted with the school principal, Mrs. Ward, and her big paddle with multiple holes drilled into it. If she wasn't threatening to discipline me with it, she was actually swatting my behind with it to discipline me.

One experience that especially stood out happened in third grade. As class started, the teacher would make me sit out in the hall for the rest of the day. I wasn't sure why. This happened every day for several weeks until my parents found out about it. During a meeting with Mrs. Ward and my teacher, my parents were told I was extremely distracting in class. They said I would talk to the other students and act out in obnoxious ways while the teacher was trying to teach. When it was time to get work done, however, I'd stare out the windows.

My authoritarian father ruled with a strong fist. Once we got home, I got a good beating and was grounded. But no matter the punishment, it didn't seem to change my behavior. I also remembered that during those years, I'd been known as "the fastest mouth in the West," as I was very friendly and liked to talk to anyone and everyone. My parents would actually brag about that to their friends. But it was also something that got me into trouble.

Recalling these past experiences made me consider trying another medication. Jill TeaSmith, my therapist, was very influential in convincing me to work with Cathy on a new medication, and I left their offices with a prescription for Depakote. After filling it, I read the many side effects written in tiny print on the bottle: nausea, vomiting, extreme drowsiness, dizziness, weakness, abdominal pain, stomach upset, rash, diarrhea, increased appetite, pain, tremor, weight gain, back pain, hair loss, headache, fever, loss of appetite, constipation, and double/blurred vision.

So nothing to worry about, I thought with heavy sarcasm.

After being on this new medication for several days, I was at work when I had the most surreal experience. I could focus on one thing at a time. This had never, ever happened to me before. Usually, I notice everything at once, every movement and every sound. When I'm talking in a meeting, I can hear the whirring of the air conditioning. I perceive the jiggling of the guy's leg next to me as he slightly bounces it under the table. I notice the guy who repeatedly clears his throat during my presentation. I notice every time anyone walks by the room. I can hear the pen moving against the paper as someone takes notes. The clicking of fingers against keyboards is constant. It's all happening at once, and I notice it all.

It was just the way my mind worked until that day. I specifically remember holding a pencil and focusing intently on it. It was the only thing I saw, and I was able to focus clearly just on it, on the bright yellow color and the details of its ridges and pointy tip. How remarkable!

A colleague stopped by my office for a quick conversation. By the end of it, she was looking at me strangely. "Anything wrong, David?" I didn't know what she was talking about. This repeatedly happened throughout the afternoon, with each conversation ending with one version or another of, "You okay?" My boss stopped by and said, "You're acting like you're in slow motion."

"Is that a bad thing?" I asked, honestly confused.

She scrunched her forehead and twisted her lips. "Well, I hope it's not a permanent thing!"

Over the next months, my boss's frustration continued to grow. My sales numbers were in rapid decline. I was no longer the kick-ass salesman I used to be.

Three months later, I was at a family party. Things were going well, or so I thought, until one of my relatives approached. "What's wrong with you today?" he asked. I quickly got defensive. This person was known for saying whatever he thought, and I wasn't in the mood.

"There's nothing wrong with me. What exactly do you mean?"

He didn't hold back. "You're so blasé! And you used to be funny. You're not funny anymore!" He wiggled the paper plate he was holding close to my face. "This plate I'm holding has more personality than you do now."

Wow. That was a wake-up call. Between that and the slump I was in at work, I knew I needed to fix things and fast.

The next day I went cold turkey off the Depakote medicine. Several weeks later, I had an appointment with Jill, my therapist, and I told her about the encounter with my relative and that I'd stopped taking the medicine.

"David! It's very dangerous to stop cold turkey off that medication!" After getting no reaction from me, she asked, "How are you feeling right now?"

"Never better," I said, and I meant it.

I spent years working closely with Jill. I have immense respect for this smart, confident therapist, and she helped to unravel many of my issues that were so deeply embedded from my past. I know that without this work—and it was hard work—I would never have been in a place where I could have met and felt worthy of a woman like Carla. I'll forever be grateful for that.

But we never did see eye-to-eye on the ADHD issue. I always believed there had to be a better way to manage it than through toxic medications with terrible side effects, or a pill that, if I accidentally took too much of it, would kill me. This simply couldn't be the answer. At least not for me. I wish someone had thought to ask about my diet during these years. Instead, the first line of defense was always to medicate.

I know there are times when medication for ADD/ADHD is necessary and helpful. I know parents who tried everything else they could, but it wasn't until they added the proper medication in the proper amount that their child was able to function in a balanced way. I would never judge these situations. I can only judge my own, and from personal experience, medication was not the answer for me.

I no longer consider my ADHD to be a negative thing. It is not a mental illness, and it is not a debilitating setback in my life. It is a strength. It took years for me to find a natural way to mitigate the negative aspects of ADHD and celebrate the positive aspects of this fantastic gift, but I did it.

Since then, I have frequently had the opportunity to lecture at various universities to business school students. There is one thing I never fail to do during my speeches. I always ask, "By a raise of hands, how many of you have been diagnosed with ADD or ADHD?" Most of the time, almost half the class will lift their hands in the air. I then tell these amazing individuals that they've been given an awesome gift. "My ADHD has been my superpower," I tell them. "I urge you to research how many famous and successful people, especially in the sciences and the arts, had these same diagnoses."

Many times, these students approach me afterward and thank me, sharing that I am the very first person in their life who has framed their diagnosis positively. They leave seeing themselves, and their potential, in a whole new way.

CHAPTER 7

THE THIRD TIME'S A CHARM

Back to Fall 2016 and my ongoing search for cancer relief...

I'd woken early this morning and crept out of bed so as not to wake Carla. I watched the sun slowly rise through my office windows, feeling great trepidation mixed with anxious hope at the thought of the difficult day ahead.

I hadn't slept well the night before. Fear of the unknown is difficult for someone like me, who works so hard at being in control. Today was also the first day of the cycling race I was supposed to compete in at the Utah Huntsman Senior games. I was disappointed to miss the cycling hill climb event I'd trained so hard for, but if it meant getting to work with a urologist oncologist who could get my bladder cancer under control, I was willing to make the trade. I planned to join the games a day late and participate in other events.

My sixtieth birthday was two months away. We'd sold our company several weeks ago; Carla had insisted we do so in order to focus on battling my cancer. I'd found that not having a job to go to every day was very challenging for me. I'd taken over all preparation for the whole juicing diet protocol, which took several hours daily, but I was having a hard time staying occupied. To help me not go crazy, I'd started riding my road bike more than ever.

I was still battling the ever-present brain fog from all the anesthesia I'd experienced during the last three surgeries. I don't understand why, but my short-term memory is severely compromised for up to a year after any surgery involving general anesthesia. This not only affected me, but it was also really hard on everyone around me—my wife, my son, Skyler, who was my business partner, my executive team—my family and friends alike struggled with this consequence of my health battles. Now here I was, facing yet another surgery in the next couple of weeks. It was hard not to feel absolute dread.

I forced my attention away from the beauty of the morning sunrise to get ready for the day. My appointment was at 2:00. I planned to drive to the Senior Games afterward, a four-hour trip, and needed to get packed. Plus, I had to do all my juicing prep and wanted to squeeze in a bike ride. It was time to get going if I were to fit it all in.

I drove to my appointment on autopilot, thoughts running like ticker tape through my mind. Would the doctor have strong opinions about chemotherapy? Would he find just the one cancerous tumor, or would there be more? Did I have any permanent brain damage from the anesthesia? I saw Carla as I rounded the corner from the elevator. We'd driven separately since she wasn't going to the games afterward. Somehow, she'd beaten me there, as she usually did. I waved to her, and she met me at the counter to check in and start the whole paperwork process yet again, a redundant task I had really grown to despise.

It was a full forty-five minutes later that I finally got called back. If only I could get back all the time I'd spent hanging out in waiting rooms! The exam room was tightly packed with cabinets and countertops, and there were pictures of kidneys, the bladder, and a prostate on the wall. The nurse was starting to ask me some follow-up questions when the doctor and his assistant walked in.

He greeted us with a broad smile that went clear to his eyes. "Hello! I'm Dr. Bishoff," he said, heartily shaking our hands. I was immediately put at ease. His whole demeanor exuded friendly confidence. He was neither too young nor too old, and his dark hair had just the right amount of gray in it. He was wearing the traditional white lab coat and sported a stethoscope around his neck.

He leaned against the exam table, and his face turned serious. "David." He looked at me. "Did you know that the number-one cause of bladder cancer is cycling?"

My eyes got big, and I looked at Carla, horrified. How did he even know I was a cyclist? "Are you serious?" I sputtered. At his wide grin, I realized how ridiculous that was, but he'd totally gotten me!

"I'm just pulling your leg!" he quipped. He pointed to my actual legs. "I just noticed the tell-tale cycling tan line you've got there." I looked down and realized that my shorts revealed the edge of the white line imprinted by many miles of cycling in the sun.

Carla and I looked at each other and laughed. We both immediately liked Dr. Bishoff. A sense of humor is high on my list of important characteristics, and I was so appreciative that he had immediately deflated any tension in the room with his prank. "My friend Walt—you gave him eight more years to live—wanted me to tell you hi," I told him.

He smiled in response and asked me to give him an abbreviated version of my cancer journey. After listening to my response and looking through my paperwork, he said, "You are producing a lot of tumors over an eighteen-month period. That is very concerning." He looked up at me, and I nodded somberly in agreement. "Let me give you my recommendation for your next surgery. But first, I need to tell you about a unique technology we have. It's called Blue Light Cystoscopy. It can diagnose tumors in the bladder using a special blue light that turns the cancer cells bright pink or red. This allows me to see your existing tumors, as well as other tumors that are in very early stages that the eye cannot see."

"That's very interesting," I responded. "Is the procedure invasive?" I'd been invaded enough to last me a lifetime!

He shrugged. "It's pretty much the same process you've had with your other surgeries: We'll put the tools, light, and camera through the urethra so they can work in the bladder. Once that procedure is done, we will remove any tumors that are found."

I glanced at Carla to read her body language while he was talking. She was leaning forward with her elbows resting on her knees, obviously listening intently. I sighed, knowing exactly what the process he'd just described felt like, and asked another question. "How long does it take for the surgery with the blue light protocol?"

He rubbed his chin and responded. "During pre-surgery, we will put a solution in your bladder. It needs to be in there for an hour. After that, the actual bladder surgery takes about sixty to ninety minutes. The surgery starts with the blue light protocol that exposes any cancer, and then we finish by removing all the tumors that are found. It's pretty straightforward." As he talked, I crossed my legs, trying not to imagine the pain I knew I would endure during recovery.

"How soon can we do this? Especially since I know I have at least one tumor growing in there."

"You'll need to stop by the front desk and talk to our scheduling person." Dr. Bishoff stood up. "I'm looking forward to helping you beat this cancer," he said.

"Not nearly as much as we are!" I declared.

Carla and I stopped at the scheduling desk. They had an opening for the following week. We walked down to the elevator hand-in-hand, smiling at each other. We both felt a sense of relief we hadn't felt in a very long time.

During the four-hour drive to St. George, I reflected on my cancer. We had been told in the past that once you get bladder cancer, there was no cure for it. I'd since researched this myself. I'd discovered something interesting. The American Cancer Society relies on information from the SEER* database, maintained by the National Cancer Institute (NCI), to provide survival statistics for different types of cancer. This database tracks five-year relative survival rates for bladder cancer in the United States, based on how far the cancer has spread. It does not, however, group cancer by AJCC TNM stages (Stage 1, Stage 2, Stage 3, etc.). Instead, it groups cancers into localized, regional, and distant stages. Here's a quick explanation of what those words mean:

- **Localized:** There is no sign that the cancer has spread outside of the bladder.
- **Regional:** The cancer has spread from the bladder to nearby structures or lymph nodes.
- **Distant:** The cancer has spread to distant parts of the body such as the lungs, liver, or bones.

Since my cancer to date had been localized, the SEER database showed that people diagnosed with bladder cancer between 2009 and 2015 had a 70% survival rate.

There are two ways to look at that: I have a 70% chance of survival or a 30% chance of dying. Dr. Bishoff gave us a confident 100% chance of survival. It was part of this cancer expert's strategy: to build a foundation of optimism that would lead to the path of remission. We had walked out of that room with renewed confidence that we would beat this cancer.

I arrived at the Huntsman Senior Games with optimism, excited to compete in the remaining three events of the cycling races. I medaled in all the events I was able to compete in, and even though I missed the first day of competition to meet with Dr. Bishoff, I had enough points from the three medals to win overall for my age group. Now, if I could only win the gold medal for beating the bladder cancer that was still growing and threatening to shorten my life!

The rest of the week flew by, and before I knew it, we were sitting in Dr. Bishoff's office again. Surprisingly, his surgical center was not at the hospital. He had a state-of-the-art facility with the specialized equipment for the blue light protocol built in his offices. Carla was concerned about the amount of anesthesia that would be used for the procedure. I was concerned because my brother was coming for a fishing trip in a couple of days, and I wanted to be coherent enough to go.

My name was called, and I looked at Carla. "Here we go again," I said. I took a deep breath and tried to calm myself down. I changed into the hospital gown, and we were led to a room where Dr. Bishoff placed a catheter in my urethra so the solution could be inserted into my bladder.

I now had to wait for an hour with my full bladder for surgery. An hour has never seemed longer to me in my entire life. I kept trying not to think about the bathroom just a few steps down the hall, where immediate relief was waiting. Then my wandering mind would think about water flowing from the bathroom faucet, and my kidneys, if such a thing were possible, would wince in pain. It got worse as the minutes ticked by, and I was gritting my teeth every time my bladder wanted to release.

I watched the time on my iPhone for the last five minutes, which ticked by in slow motion, sweating now in pain. As the clock finally turned over the hour, a nurse came in and told me I could go to the bathroom. I practically ran down the hall. The nurse was waiting for me when I was done.

"Let's go to the surgical room," she instructed. "They're waiting for you there."

I looked at her in surprise. "Doesn't an anesthesiologist meet with my wife and me first?"

She shook her head. "Everything is done in the surgical room, so the anesthesiologist will meet you in there." This concerned Carla because she wanted to talk to that person first. She wanted to make sure they knew that I am a lightweight when it comes to anesthesia. Unfortunately, they didn't give her that chance.

I gave Carla a hug and kiss goodbye, and the nurse led me back to the surgical room. When she opened the door, I was greeted by three nurses. Dr. Bishoff was not in the room yet, but they introduced me to the anesthesiologist, who was sitting to the left of the exam table. I'd been through all of this enough times now that I thought I knew what to expect. I got myself situated on the table in the most modest way possible, extra aware of all the females in the room. Two of the nurses started prepping me, which meant that they uncovered me up to my chest, and I was totally exposed. I just closed my eyes and tried to imagine I was somewhere—anywhere—else.

With three female nurses standing at the end of the table with a straight shot to my privates, the anesthesiologist prepared my left wrist area for an IV. After a few moments of pain from his poking around, he grunted as if put out about something. Since my antenna was on high alert, I raised my head and asked him what was wrong. He looked at me with annoyance. "Your vein has blown," he accused as if it was my fault. "I have to start over somewhere else." I looked from him to the nurses in exasperation. In all my surgeries over the years, this was the first time I'd blown a vein. But it wasn't the last—somehow, three veins blew before he was able to administer the IV. I'm pretty sure I could've done better at finding my own vein one-handed. But finally, blissfully, everything went dark.

After the surgery, Dr. Bishoff came in with a big smile. Carla, anxious for a report, quickly asked, "How did the procedure go?"

He sat down and put both hands on his knees. "We found a total of four tumors and a nodule that we removed from the prostate." Carla and I looked at each other, eyebrows raised in surprise. Still quite groggy, I was finding it difficult to put words together, so Carla did the talking for us.

"What is the nodule that you found?" she asked.

"A prostate nodule is a firm, knuckle-like area on the prostate gland. A nodule can develop due to a variety of reasons, including prostatitis and prostate cancer. At this point, we have to wait for lab results to see if it is non-cancerous." Not waiting for a response, he dove into the four cancerous tumors that he'd found in my bladder. "Two of the tumors I could see with my eyes, and the other two tumors were revealed by the blue light. That means, had I not used the blue light procedure, those two tiny tumors that I could not see would not have been removed. Then at your next cystoscopy in three months, I would see those tumors, and you would have had to have another surgery."

I closed my eyes and tried to process the mix of emotions I was feeling at that news.

Looking from Carla to me, he said, "With your bladder cancer history and the results from today, I am recommending that you do two rounds of BCG."

I had enough cognitive awareness to ask, "What is BCG?"

Rubbing his chin with his right hand, he explained, "Bacillus Calmette-Guerin, or BCG, is the most common intravesical immunotherapy for treating early-stage bladder cancer. It's used to help keep the cancer from growing and to help keep it from coming back. BCG is a germ that's related to the one that causes tuberculosis." Although I was still fairly out of it, I realized what all those words meant, and my heart sunk. *No, please not chemo.* I had been praying and doing absolutely everything I could to avoid chemotherapy. Things became even foggier, and my head dropped to my hands.

"You better get him home to sleep off the anesthesia," Dr. Bishoff instructed Carla. I don't really remember going home and getting into bed. But once I was awake and fairly cognizant, Carla recounted the rest of what Dr. Bishoff said after the surgery.

He was adamant that I had to do the BCG if I wanted to exterminate the bladder cancer. Carla said that we asked Dr. Bishoff what he would do if he were in my position. He didn't hesitate in his response. "If I had gone through three surgeries to remove twenty-one tumors over eighteen months and wanted to save my bladder, I would do the BCG," he affirmed. "I'd do two rounds: six weeks on, six weeks off, and six weeks on, to get rid of it. If it were me, that's what I would do."

Carla knew I was determined to avoid chemo, and she understood why. Everyone we knew who'd undergone chemo had been absolutely wrecked by it. It was no way to live. We even knew people who had died not from their cancer but from the effects of the chemo. She explained that to Dr. Bishoff.

He responded that if we kept doing what we'd been doing and cutting away at these tumors every time, he'd eventually have to take my bladder out. He also explained that this particular chemotherapy doesn't kill the immune system. It needs a strong immune system to work. Basically, they're putting tuberculosis in your bladder to teach the immune system how to attack it. That way, you not only get rid of the cancer, but it never comes back because the body has learned how to kill the cancer cells on its own.

"So I need your immune system to be ramped up for this to work," he wrapped up.

After Carla refreshed my memory about this discussion, all I could say was, "Let me think about it."

I got up the next morning despite the post-surgery pain and did the juicing protocol like I always did. I spent the two hours it took to prep it mulling over what Dr. Bishoff had said and what had transpired over the last eighteen months. Two things were bugging me. First, why wasn't this cancer-busting juicing protocol working? I had followed the juicing diet now for ten months. I hadn't discussed it with Dr. Bishoff at all; he'd never asked any questions about my diet, and he seemed fairly medicine-focused like most doctors I knew. But I didn't want to give up on it yet; I was stubborn and had committed to myself that I would do it for two years. My competitive nature wanted to see it through.

The second question plaguing me was whether I should relent and proceed with the BCG despite my tremendous fears. I trusted this doctor, and he insisted that I would have to have my bladder removed if I did not do the BCG. There was no way that I wanted to have a urostomy pouch for the rest of my life. At this point, doing the BCG was the lesser of two evils, which felt so discouraging. I had worked so hard on my diet to boost my immune system to fight the cancer. Now my heart and mind felt like I had no choice but to agree to the treatment. Later that day, I reluctantly told Carla I was ready to schedule the BCG.

Talk about a crazy time in our life. I was able to go on the fishing trip with my brother after surgery and enjoyed it despite the inevitable pain from recovery. Then Carla threw me an amazing surprise sixtieth birthday and retirement party with all of our closest family and friends. It was a meaningful milestone that I'll never forget. Meanwhile, Carla was pushing hard for us to move from our home. Through a fluke, we'd had our house tested for radon and discovered we'd unknowingly been living in a home for twelve years with high levels of radon gas coming through the foundation. She thought this might be a cause of my cancer and was aggressively hunting to downsize our home and move. All of this kept us very busy.

A note from Carla about radon:

Radon gas is produced during the natural breakdown of radioactive elements in soils and rocks. It is radioactive and has no taste, smell, or color. Even though it's a natural gas that comes from the earth, it can be toxic.

During the time that we were battling David's cancer, a friend mentioned to us that since our house was built on granite rock, we should have it tested for radon. A safe radon level is anything under four. Our home tested at twenty-nine! Evidently, our home was very well-built; we loved that it was so energy efficient. But this also meant that there was no way for the gas to escape. We were living in an airtight vacuum that sucked the gas through the foundation and the floor. We immediately hired a company who came in and drilled through the cement foundation and placed pipes that pumped the gas out through the top of the roof.

We tested for radon again, and although the numbers had dropped, our levels were still elevated. We had a second pipe system installed. Meanwhile, I read an article that said radon gas was the second-leading cause of lung disease. That gave me serious pause. Every doctor we went to that didn't already know David always asked, "Are you a smoker?" He'd say no, but that his dad had been, so he'd been exposed to secondhand smoke. Evidently, smoking was linked to bladder cancer as well as lung cancer. Perhaps radon was linked to both as well? Could that explain why David kept getting these tumors?

We tested our levels again, and we were still above the safe zone. I'd already wanted to move to be closer to my grandkids, and this just motivated me even more. I'll never have any proof that this contributed to his bladder cancer, but I sure feel like it did. Radon is a toxin. Everything we are trying to do to stay healthy is based on getting rid of toxins through proper nutrition and lifestyle and eliminating exposure to toxins as much as possible.

We had a third company install a radon removal system, and they guaranteed the radon would never go above a four. It's now probably one of the safest homes in the area, but I'd made up my mind, and we moved off the mountain.

David

A few days later, we got a personal call from Dr. Bishoff saying that the results came back from the lab on the nodule, and they were negative: not cancer. This was really great news. Now it was on to the chemo I had dreaded for so long. I scheduled the eighteen-week BCG protocol. Starting in November, I would go in once a week for six weeks, take a six-week break, and then have another round of treatments over the next six weeks.

Chemo was one of the most difficult things I've ever had to endure. Every Wednesday, I had my bladder injected with tuberculosis. The nurse wore a special protective bodysuit, thick rubber gloves, and a glass shield over her face. I tried to joke with her a bit, hoping to release some tension. "Wow, you look prepared for serious chemical warfare!" I quipped nervously. She simply smiled and said, "We could get tuberculosis if any of this gets on us." So much for my nerves. At home, I had to have my own bathroom because the output from my bladder after treatment was dangerous enough it could kill someone.

At my first appointment, the technician told me what to expect. "You will experience quite a bit of pain. There will also be bleeding. The pain and bleeding will get worse with each treatment as we aggravate the bladder and force the immune system to fight the cancer cells."

She wasn't lying. Even with all that I'd endured with this whole bladder cancer journey so far, this was excruciating, and every week it got worse. When I got home after each treatment, I'd spend hours rolling from my back to side, to stomach, to other side, following instructions to ensure the chemo was applied correctly to my bladder. I was miserable and completely unable to do anything for four to five days after each treatment. Most people don't finish two full rounds of BCG treatment. It's simply too hard. Dr. Bishoff wanted me to do two but told me if I had to quit, they understood. Because of my belief in this doctor, I did the treatments even when I didn't want to.

After just the second treatment, I told Carla I didn't think I'd be able to do this. I couldn't take it. She said she completely understood and supported me in whatever I decided to do. I know that as my caretaker, it was very hard for her to helplessly watch me repeatedly suffer.

This became the pattern. I'd go get injected on Wednesday and then wanted to die until Monday. By Tuesday, I'd feel a little better. I'd dig deep and decide to do one more treatment. Then on Wednesday, it would start all over again. But as predicted, the suffering intensified each time.

Chemo becomes your life. You can't do anything. You can't make plans. It is all you do. I was so grateful for the six-week break between rounds, but the second round was far worse than the first. Each week, I told Carla that I could not finish, and each week she told me she understood. Part of her probably wanted me to quit because my suffering was so hard for her to watch. But somehow, by every Tuesday night, I'd decide that I would go in for just one more treatment.

On March 29th, 2017, I finished the last of the twelve doses of BCG. I had done it. I don't know how, but I'd survived. I walked out of Dr. Bishoff's office that day, so relieved to know I had no more treatments to endure.

We'd had so many miracles throughout this cancer battle. It was a miracle that we'd found Dr. Bishoff and were able to get in to see him so quickly. It was a miracle that I was able to finish all twelve of the brutal chemo treatments. Now we were praying for the biggest miracle of all, the miracle we'd wanted all along: no more tumors. At my check-up three months later, I needed to be cancer-free.

CHAPTER 8

OH NO! NOT SLEEP APNEA, TOO!

"He'd been snoring incessantly!" Susan declared, elbowing her husband, John, good-naturedly. We were out to dinner with some good friends, and the conversation had turned to sleep issues as we ate our salads. "Neither of us were able to get a good night's sleep with all that racket going on! He snores so loudly he even wakes himself up!"

"It's true," John agreed, setting down his fork. "It was time to do something about it, so I got a referral to see a sleep medicine specialist."

I glanced at Carla, who was looking at me pointedly. She'd been complaining about my terrible snoring for years now. John went on to explain that actually booking the appointment was a bit hard on his ego, as the whole concept made him feel old. "But Dr. Staheli, the specialist, was really great," he went on. "He is personable and has a great bedside manner—which comes in handy for a sleep specialist!" he quipped.

Dr. Staheli had advised John to do a sleep study. This entailed an overnight stay at a clinic where he would be hooked up with lots of electrodes that would monitor his body and brain while he slept.

"Was it weird to have a nurse watch you sleep all night?" I asked him, shuddering a bit at the thought.

"Yes, it was weird, and I almost backed out of it, but Susan 'strongly encouraged' me to follow through," he said, giving her a meaningful look. We all laughed, knowing how that must have gone down. Surprised, I realized I had finished my salad and had not even remembered eating it, I was listening so intently. I was intrigued by the story because it hit home. Over the past couple of years, I had started waking myself up with loud snores followed by a sensation that I was choking. It was scary and disconcerting. At this point, Carla chimed in.

"So how'd it go?" she asked. "David's snoring keeps me up a lot, too."

We paused while the waitress delivered our main courses, and then John continued his story. During the sleep study, he'd been asleep less than two hours before the nurse who was monitoring him woke him up and mandated he be placed on a CPAP. A CPAP (Continuous Positive Airway Pressure) is a breathing machine that is connected to a mask that covers the face and nose. The next morning, at the end of the study, the nurse told him that the CPAP had helped him tremendously.

His AHI,[2] or the number of "events" per hour, was almost ninety. In his case, this meant he was waking up almost ninety times per hour! That number seemed crazy to all of us. But once the CPAP had been placed, his score dropped to less than two AHI per hour. The nurse then told him there was some good news.

"What would that be?" he'd asked.

"You only have OSA, or Obstructive Sleep Apnea. It's very common and happens as we age. Luckily, you don't have Central Sleep Apnea. CSA is associated with more severe illnesses." She explained that the doctor would go over all his results at their next appointment.

At the follow-up, Dr. Staheli told John he had severe sleep apnea. A severe case is anything higher than 15 AHI per hour. At 90 AHI, he was off the charts. The doctor gave him a prescription for a CPAP, and he and Susan picked out a machine and several masks. He'd narrowed it down to two different types: one covered his mouth and nose, and the other just covered his nose. He liked the nose mask best, he explained, because he is a nose breather at night. He laughed and added, "It's not the sexiest thing, that's for sure!"

---

2 AHI (Apnea Hypopnea Index) refers to the classifications of sleep apnea. Specifically, AHI refers to the number of apneas and/or hypopneas per hour of sleep (or study time). The index number reflects the severity of sleep apnea.

AHI: < 5	Normal Range
AHI: 5 to <15	Mild Sleep Apnea
AHI: 15 to <30	Moderate Sleep Apnea
AHI: > or = to 30	Severe Sleep Apnea

I looked at Susan. "How is the CPAP working for you?" I asked her.

"I'm in love!" she effused. "I can finally get a good night's sleep!"

Laughing, I turned to John. "So it's worth it? What has the CPAP done for you?"

His response was immediate. "It's made all the difference. When I wake up in the morning, I finally feel completely rested. I used to be so tired all the time! Before the CPAP, I was falling asleep in the late afternoon."

John and Susan were both smiling, and I looked over to Carla to see what was going on. She was giving me *that* look.

"What's that look for?" I challenged, even though I already knew the answer.

Smiling sweetly, she said, "You should go see John's doctor and see if they will do a sleep study on you." I was actually kind of interested at that point, but I wasn't ready to admit it. I just shrugged her comment off and finished up my salmon. Oh, the pride and ego of David Meine!

As the days (and nights) passed, I was more aware than ever of my crappy sleep patterns. I still struggled with snoring and waking to the sensation of choking, and it scared me more than ever now that I knew what it possibly meant. Plus, my pervasive fears about my constant brain fog persisted, and I wondered if my memory issues might be tied to sleep apnea. I kept thinking about how enthusiastic both John and Susan were and how good he said he felt. *If he was willing to do a sleep study, then why shouldn't I?* I finally told myself. I texted John and asked for Dr. Staheli's contact information.

The doctor was booked out for months, but I made an appointment with his physician assistant. After she reviewed my paperwork, she strongly recommended I do a sleep study. That left me with mixed feelings: I really did not want to find out that I needed to be hooked up to a machine to breathe at night, but I also knew I really needed to solve my sleep problem.

After I got home and told Carla about the appointment (and tried to ignore her pleased smile when she learned I'd actually scheduled the sleep study), I went straight to the internet to do some research. Here is just a little of what I found:

> Left untreated, sleep apnea can have serious and life-shortening consequences: high blood pressure, heart disease, stroke, automobile accidents caused by falling asleep at the wheel, diabetes, depression, and other ailments.[3]

That was incredibly reassuring, I thought sarcastically. Searching further, I found more on the John Hopkins Center for Sleep website:

> You've probably heard that regular exercise and a heart-healthy diet are the most important things you can do for your cardiovascular health. As it turns out,

3 TrueTox Laboratories, LLC, "Opiates & Sleep," 2019, *https://www.truetoxlabs.com/opiates-sleep/.*

> though, the quality of sleep you receive is also critical to your heart's wellbeing.[4]

In particular, undiagnosed sleep apnea is directly tied to an increased risk in cardiovascular and metabolic health. The scariest part? You might not even know you have this very common problem.

Reading further in the article, they described the two forms of sleep apnea. First, there is obstructive sleep apnea (OSA), which happens when air can't flow into or out of the nose or mouth, although you're trying to breathe. Second, there is central sleep apnea (CSA), which happens when the brain fails to send the right signals to your muscles to make you start breathing. This type is less common and can be considered more dangerous. I remembered that John had been diagnosed with OSA, the more common form. I was hoping with all of my being that I had neither one of these conditions.

The night of my sleep study, I felt nervous. Carla tried her best to be sympathetic, but I knew she was really looking forward to a good night's sleep without me waking her up with my snoring. It was dark when I arrived at the sleep center at 9 p.m. A nurse led me through a honey-colored door into what turned out to be a bedroom. It was neat, clean, and featured a queen-sized bed. The walls were painted a cream color, and there were pictures of nature around the room. To the right of the bed was a tall dresser. A computer-like device sat on a rolling metal tray in front of the dresser, with lots of wires coming out of it.

---

4 "The Dangers of Uncontrolled Sleep Apnea," 17 June 2021, *https://www.hopkinsmedicine.org/health/wellness-and-prevention/the-dangers-of-uncontrolled-sleep-apnea.*

The nurse asked me to lift my shirt so she could start attaching the electrode pads to my chest, stomach, and arms. She then had me lie on the bed face up so she could attach some electrodes to my head. After rechecking everything, she asked, "Are you comfortable?"

"I only sleep with a sheet at night. Can we take these off?" I pointed to the heavier blankets. "Also, I can't have anything touching my feet." She gave me an odd look at that one, so I explained quickly about my peripheral neuropathy.

She worked to get me comfortable while describing what would happen. "I will be monitoring your signal output for several hours. If it appears that you have sleep apnea, I will put you on a CPAP machine. Don't worry…" She stopped and looked in my eyes, sensing I was nervous, "Just try to get a good night's sleep." With that, she flipped off the lights and shut the door, leaving me alone with my electrodes.

I had no idea how a good night would be possible with all these wires attached to me, sleeping in a strange bed in a strange place, and not next to Carla! I started counting backward from a hundred, a technique that sometimes helped me to fall asleep, but it didn't work. I did some breathing exercises, and that slowly helped my mind and body to relax. After that, I started counting backward again and finally fell into a fitful sleep.

Sometime during the night, I became aware that the nurse was working on me. When I opened my eyes, she said, "Everything is okay. I just need to put a mask on you." I fell back to sleep, and I don't really remember anything else. At six o'clock in the morning, I woke up. A different nurse came in. She was tall, skinny, and all business as she started taking off the electrodes. I asked her what they found out during the night, and she said that I would have to wait until the doctor got the report. That was a big letdown for me. I really struggle to be patient about test results.

I just smiled and asked how long it would take to hear back. "You'll need to set up an appointment with Dr. Judd, who'll be handling your case." I followed her to the nurse's station, where we set up an appointment for the following week. She then pulled out a clipboard and asked me to complete a one-page post-sleep questionnaire. It didn't take very long to fill it out, and I handed it back and wished her a happy holiday season. (See Post-Sleep Questionnaire in Appendix I.)

Walking out to my car in the still-dark sky, I felt like I was totally in the dark about this whole sleep apnea business. Carla was just getting up when I got home. She asked, "How did your sleep test go?" I spoke over my shoulder as I walked into the bathroom and said it went well but that we would have no results for another week. "Bummer," she said. Patience is not the strongest suit for either of us. We like to get things done, and the waiting and not knowing are painful for us both.

Because we were in the midst of the holiday season, it was easy for me to get distracted. Carla and I both love the holidays, and the Christmas season is always special with our large family. The week flew by and, before I knew it, I was on my way back to the sleep center for my appointment with the doctor. This time around, it was daylight, and snow was gently falling. I felt optimistic, my spirits boosted by the beauty of it all.

Dr. Judd introduced himself when he came into the waiting room. "Hello, David, how are you doing today?" he asked, shaking my hand.

"I'll let you know after our meeting," I deadpanned.

"We have never lost a patient here in the sleep center," he returned. I gave an obligatory laugh and thought, *That was almost funny.* We walked into his office, a tiny space barely big enough for his little desk. I sat and started leafing through a pamphlet on sleep disorders as he pulled up the report on his computer. There was a lot of information to review (See Sleep Study Results Form in Appendix I). "So, David, looking over your sleep study, it shows that you have two forms of sleep apnea." I looked up quickly from the pamphlet, my good mood immediately disintegrating into one of consternation and frustration. He could tell I was shocked by the news and looked to head me off.

"Look, I know that wasn't what you wanted to hear, but the good news is, now that we know what you're dealing with, there is really great technology available that will help you control it. You're going to feel a lot better. Here, take a look at this page," he offered, handing me a paper from the results report (see Appendix I). "Your AHI was at 82.5 before we put the first CPAP machine and mask on you." From what I'd learned from my friend John's sleep test, I knew that 82.5 was extremely high.

We discussed the midnight event, where the nurse had come into the room and put me on a CPAP machine. I noticed that my oxygen levels at that time were going down into the eighties, which was not good. Then the doctor pointed out on another page of the report that my oxygen had gone into the sixties, which is dangerous. At 2 a.m., the tech came back in and switched me to a BiPAP machine. Seeing the reality of it all on paper blew me away.

"Why did I have to be put on a different machine?" I asked him.

"Your CSA is all about your brain not telling your lungs to inflate, which causes you to choke. When that happens, the brain kicks back in and tells the lungs to inflate. These events cause very poor sleep quality. The BiPAP pushes air in to inflate the lungs and monitors that you are breathing out. We set it to certain parameters to keep you in an even state of breathing."

I set the report on my lap and brought my hands to my face, putting my index fingers on either side of the bridge of my nose in an effort to calm myself. It all just felt like too much, and I was very discouraged. I had just finished chemotherapy for my bladder cancer nine months ago. Now I was getting this diagnosis right in the middle of the holiday season. I wanted to say a big, fat "bah humbug" to this news. The doctor was still talking, explaining the ins and outs of the BiPAP machine. I listened halfheartedly. He handed me a prescription and said the IHC Home Care Equipment personnel would help me with the BiPAP and mask selection.

About a week later, I was sitting in a chair at the IHC Home Care Center, watching the technician pull out several masks. Mentally, I started picturing myself as a fighter pilot, having to gear up in all sorts of uncomfortable contraptions just to try and sleep each night. This image really is a pretty accurate depiction of how I was feeling about the whole mask situation.

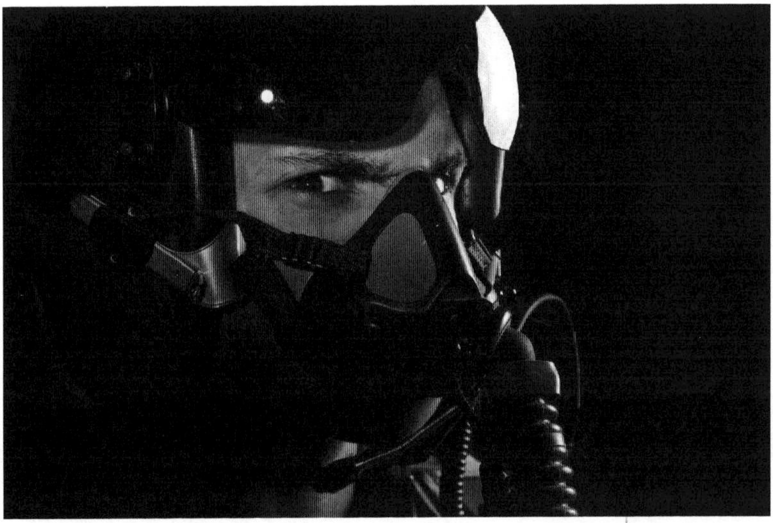

I was fitted with a mask and sent home with my new BiPAP machine. I followed all of the instructions for setting up the equipment and filled up the reservoir with the required distilled water. By 10:30 p.m., our usual bedtime, I was prepared for my first night's sleep, hooked up to my strange new apparatus.

Sitting on the edge of the bed, I pulled on the mask that covered my nose and mouth. It was connected with a long hose to the rest of the machine. I pushed the "on" button, and the machine pushed a burst of cool air into my mask. I looked at Carla and smiled but didn't know if she could see it under all that. I knew she was excited to see how this all worked out and was hoping to wake up tomorrow morning after an uninterrupted sleep—we both were! I laid back on the bed and started the process of falling asleep.

The next thing I knew, I woke up about eight hours later. While stretching in bed, I realized that I still had the mask on. I reached over and turned off the BiPAP and pulled off the mask. Carla was already awake and waiting for me to wake up. "Well, how do you feel?" she queried.

Pausing for a few moments to inventory how I felt, I said, "Surprisingly, I really feel rested."

She responded with a huge smile, "I got a great night's sleep also."

After that first night, I tried several different masks. I ended up settling on a nasal mask, like the one in this photo.

I've found there is a pattern with my health struggles: Although the initial diagnosis can be really overwhelming, once I know with certainty what the problem is and I'm able to find viable solutions, I feel empowered. I feel relief. Yes, it was tough to take the news of my severe CSA initially, but once I realized there was nothing I could do to force my brain to tell my lungs to inflate while sleeping, I was all in for the solution. I wanted to feel better and fully understood that sleep is the foundation of good health.

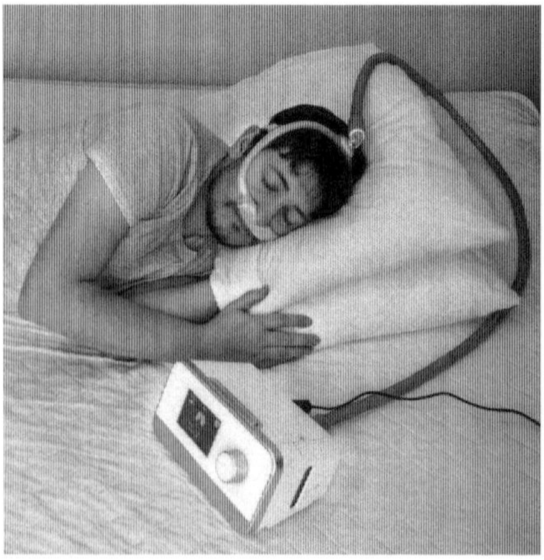

Since that December night back in 2017 when I first used it, I have not missed using my BiPAP even one time. Every time I go on vacation or travel out of town, I pack it all up and take it with me. I made a commitment to myself that even if it made me look like an old man, my quality of life was more important. Even if I go to bed each night looking like a fighter pilot, I'll do it. I want to live to be ninety-five years old, with vibrant health and mental clarity. I want to celebrate my fiftieth wedding anniversary with Carla, throwing down some old-man grooves with my beautiful wife on the dance floor. A little sleep-apparatus inconvenience is worth it.

CHAPTER 9

61 YEARS OLD AND FALLING APART (MY DEPENDENCE ON NSAIDS)

To our immense relief, the cystoscopy exams in June, September, and December of 2017, and March of 2018 with Dr. Bishoff showed that no cancer tumors had manifested. At each appointment, he would smile his wide, authentic smile and say, "Everything looks great, and I believe that the bladder is totally healed."

My whole focus in life from April 2015 until March 2017 had been beating cancer. But I'd been ignoring some other problems. During the two years that I did the juicing protocol, my daily pain level had skyrocketed. I had severe pain from my peripheral neuropathy, my back pain, and severe knee arthritis (acquired from two arthroscopic surgeries years prior to treat athletic injuries). Strangely, my arthritic knee started having flare-ups during this time, and they were pretty debilitating. I was used to the pain of athletic injuries, but this was different. With my attention intensely focused on the cancer, I simply attributed the increased pain levels to what the cancer was doing to my body and kept chugging the over-the-counter pain relievers.

It never dawned on me to ask Dr. Bishoff about why my general body pain had escalated over the past three years and why the daily pain continued despite the good cancer results.

With four clean bladder scans under my belt, I felt it was time to discontinue the diet juicing protocol. I thought it had done its job in helping with the cancer battle. Soon—very soon—I would find out that this cancer-busting diet was, in fact, anything but.

In April of 2018, I had a relapse with my back pain and started physical therapy again with Rogan. My knee pain also increased, and going up and down stairs was causing extreme pain under my right knee cap. Years ago, I'd been told I needed a knee replacement, but when I met with the surgeon, I discovered I was not a candidate for surgery due to spacing between the joints.

Secretly, I'd been relieved; my friend Scott had his right knee replaced and was miserable for several months. He told me in private he was supposed to have his other knee done, but after doing the first one, no way was he going to do that surgery again. Knowing this, I asked Rogan what I should do about my knee. He suggested doing physical therapy for the knee in addition to what he was doing for my back.

It seemed that at sixty-one years old I'd become a cliché old man. I was falling apart. How had this become my life? All I knew was that having serious back issues, knee issues, and arthritis was extremely frustrating. And the ibuprofen, Lortab, and Naproxen were not working very well anymore.

A friend and I were discussing all of our physical ailments when I realized we were having the "old-man discussion;" you know, the one you heard your grandparents having years ago when you thought all they talked about was their aches and pains? That was us. We spent our hour-long lunch talking about his heart attack and balance issues and all my discouraging pain problems. As we wrapped up, he advised me to check into a local pain solution company he'd heard about.

As soon as I got to my car, I Googled and found the company he'd recommended. I read through multiple patient reviews of their alternative treatments including stem cell and platelet-rich plasma (PRP) procedures for patients with chronic pain. I was intrigued enough to fill out the information form.

NSAID Doctor #1: Meeting Dr. Khan

Long story short, this is how I met Dr. Khan. Dr. Qamar Khan is a provider at Wasatch Pain Solutions, a specialized clinic for sufferers of acute and chronic pain. We were coordinating stem cell treatment for my knee and PRP for my spine, and I was feeling optimistic. Then he caught me completely off-guard with what he said next: "We need to discuss your use of NSAIDs." (He pronounced this as N-saids.)

I looked at him blankly. "I have no idea what that word means," I responded.

"NSAIDs is an abbreviation for non-steroidal anti-inflammatory drugs, which are medications such as ibuprofen that are used to control pain and inflammation."

"Oh," I said, realizing he was talking about my go-to daily medications. "Well, I've participated in a wide variety of sports for a lot of years now, and it's definitely caught up to me. For at least the last thirty years, I've taken pain medication pretty constantly. My over-the-counter medicine of choice is Advil. My primary care physician typically prescribes Naproxen for muscle injuries and Lortab for my back when it's really killing me."

He stopped me there and asked, "How often do you take Advil or Naproxen?"

"I take 800 milligrams one to three times a day."

At this, he furrowed his brow and looked very serious. "David," he said, "for us to proceed with the treatment, you will have to stop taking any form of NSAIDs for thirty days. Additionally, you will need to stay off of them for 120 days after the treatment."

What? I thought. He might as well have told me I'd have to stop breathing air! There was no way I could survive without my pain medications. "Are you kidding me?" I asked, hoping he was somehow exaggerating.

"I am very serious," he continued. "NSAIDs interfere with the healing capabilities of the stem cells. They do this by inhibiting the stem cells' ability to regrow bone. Furthermore, residual NSAID presence in the joints may weaken bone, causing structural instability."

I was stunned. Dr. Khan could've probably knocked me over with a feather. I was both totally confused and frustrated by this news. Committing to five months of living without any of my pain medications simply didn't seem possible. The whole reason I was at this consultation was because of the extreme pain in my knee just from walking up and down the stairs in my home. I'd had to give up hiking because it was unbearable. Even walking around the neighborhood or just sitting in a chair was sometimes too painful to take. And that was *with* the pain relievers! How could I possibly do this?

I scheduled my first treatment thirty-five days away and told Dr. Khan I would keep NSAIDs out of my system, but as I left the office, I was seriously questioning my ability to make it through the next twenty-four hours, let alone the next month. Not to mention 120 days after the procedure as well.

During dinner that night, I tried to explain it all to Carla, but it was hard for me to give her a clear picture of what was going to happen. She was obviously very dubious of my ability to live without my precious pain medications and expressed her concern.

Even though I was in pain that night, I did not take my usual 800 mgs of Advil before bed. Taking the medicine dulled the aches enough that I could at least fall asleep. Tonight would be my first night without it in years. I kept telling myself that I could sacrifice NSAIDs and tolerate knee pain in the short run in order to gain no pain in my knee in the long run. But my brain balked at this pep talk, reminding me that I still had the burning pain in my feet, the sharp pain in my back, the arthritic pain in my left hand, and the shooting pain in my knee that wouldn't be medicated. My pain crutch was taken away cold turkey, and I was mentally unprepared to travel this bumpy path.

During the day, I could find distractions that helped me not dwell on the pain. But that first night, all I could think about was that there would be no relief. It was like when I had sprained my ankle on a fifty-mile hike and still had twenty miles to go. My ankle hurt so badly, but I had no choice—I had to finish the hike. I laid in bed and tried to distract my mind by counting backward from a hundred. I had to start over at least a dozen times when my thoughts were hijacked by the pain, and I knew there was no relief in sight. Finally, everything went dark, and I slept fitfully through the night.

This went on every day for the next thirty-five days. It is very difficult to live with pain. Chronic pain is directly linked to anxiety and depression, and I get why. It was super hard to stay positive and act like everything was okay. In fact, research states that back pain, cancer pain, and arthritis account for a large portion of the chronic pain conditions in people who commit suicide. I had all three of those sources of pain at once. I never became suicidal, but I'm sure I was depressed.

After those long, pain-filled thirty-five days without NSAIDs, I started the stem cell treatments and PRP protocols. I won't bore you with the details or the specifics. Suffice it to say, it was not an immediate, magical cure-all for my knee pain. Toward the end of June 2018, I was pretty miserable. At one of the treatments, I wanted to verify with Dr. Kahn that I could start back on NSAIDs at the end of September. His response left me totally discouraged.

His dark eyes stared into mine as he said, "David, I strongly recommend that you never take NSAIDs again for the rest of your life." You can imagine how deeply his recommendation shook me up.

Shocked, I couldn't help but blurt out, "How am I supposed to deal with my arthritis and neuropathy for the rest of my life without NSAIDs?"

All he could say to that was, "You will have to figure it out."

This news devastated me. Going cold turkey off the pain medicine was so difficult, I'd even started wondering if it was possible that I was addicted to NSAIDs. After all these weeks without taking them, it felt like I was having withdrawals. It also seemed I actually had increased pain and swelling.

When we started the stem cell treatment plan, I thought Dr. Khan had said I only had to be off the pain medicine for five months. That had been the lifeline I'd clung to, and I'd been counting down the days. It turns out I'd incorrectly inferred that information, and my lifeline was yanked away.

Pain was my nemesis. Over the years, I had managed to only minimally use what I thought were the truly addictive pain drugs. I only used Oxycodone, Lortab, and Naproxen for short periods of time. When I had my first back surgery, I was off those medicines six days after the surgery, surviving instead on over-the-counter stuff. I'd always congratulated myself for my self-restraint. I had a lot of fear that I would go down the rabbit hole with those drugs and ruin my life. But now, I was being told that NSAIDs, although not as bad as those addictive painkillers, were also harmful, somehow affecting my health at the cellular level.

The stem cell protocol required me to wear a hefty, black medical brace to protect my right knee for two months. Many times I thought, *All this better be worth it!* The pain in my right knee dropped dramatically each week, which kept me going, but I was in great pain everywhere else. For several weeks after my no-NSAIDs-ever-again revelation with Dr. Khan, I was pretty despondent about how I was going to manage pain for the rest of my life.

I am grateful for the relief Dr. Khan provided in my knee and eventually in my back from his therapies. He was a good doctor—great, even, in his field. But I wish he had thought to ask me some additional, holistic questions. We never discussed how my diet could be contributing to my pain or how certain foods and beverages could be causing inflammation. Instead, I had to be my own advocate and, as Dr. Khan said, "figure it out."

To be very clear, I am not anti-doctor. Even when I tell stories about the doctors that made mistakes and added to my pain, such as Dr. Frankenstein and the vein-blowing anesthesiologist, I know they were simply trying their best to do their jobs in a competent manner. I always joke with people when they share a bad medical story by saying, "That's why they call it *practicing* medicine." But even good doctors get very little training on nutrition in medical school. Instead, they prescribe, and we try to survive. I'd been struggling to survive for a long time now. As a result, I'd come to the harsh realization that I was absolutely drug-dependent, and my drug of choice was any form of NSAIDs I could get my hands on.

NSAID Doctor #2: An Introduction to Dr. Gundry

Serendipity sometimes plays a big role in my life. Toward the end of July 2018, a simple pop-up ad turned out to be very serendipitous for me. Since I don't watch the news and watch very little of anything on TV, I typically don't see a lot of advertisements. Surfing the internet or looking at social media is a whole different story, though. That's where marketing gets me. Typically, I am a big sucker for new fishing products. Make one purchase, and the marketers start throwing up ads for similar products. Today, however, for some reason, an advertisement for a podcast that was not even related to fishing came up on my internet feed.

The ad was accompanied by a picture of a Dr. Steven Gundry. With white hair, a gray beard, glasses, and a pleasant smile, he looked like a respectable grandpa, which was easy for me to relate to. The podcast was titled, *The Healthy Foods That Are Killing You.*[5] For some reason, that title intrigued me. From 2009 to 2016, Carla, my son Skyler, and I helped thousands of people get healthy with training in nutrition, exercise, meal planning, and brain training. I thought I had a pretty good idea of which foods were good for me.

Before watching Dr. Gundry's video, I looked him up on the internet. His credentials were impressive. I read that "he was a renowned cardiologist, surgeon, medical device inventor, and author. He believes every human deserves vitality and

---

5 Lewis Howes, "The Health Goods That Are Killing You," The School of Greatness Podcast, 9 August 2017, *https://lewishowes.com/podcast/h-dr-gundry/.*

longevity."[6] Another link stated, "He has worked in medicine for over forty years and now teaches people how to avoid surgery by using his unique vision of human nutrition."[7]

After reading good and bad reviews on Dr. Gundry, I decided it was in my best interest to watch the podcast. In the introduction, Lewis Howes, the interviewer (somebody famous that I had never heard of) stated, "Dr. Gundry's mission is to end disease." He then addressed Dr. Gundry and said, "You're saying that, to end disease, it starts and ends through the gut."

Dr. Gundry answered, "Yes, and that we can extend our lives based on what we eat."

I was totally intrigued by their discussion on gut health. They talked about how much the gut affects us, covering bloating, gas, cravings for carbs, low energy, brain fog, and skin issues. What really caught my interest was the discussion on bacteria. For a moment, I thought they were talking about Star Wars when they brought up mitochondria and how bacteria work together. In the Star Wars series, Midi-chlorians are microscopic, intelligent life forms that originated from the foundation of life and were especially strong with Force-sensitive beings like Luke Skywalker and Yoda. I wonder if the writers from Star Wars created Midi-chlorians based on mitochondria.

Since I had no idea what mitochondria were, I went to the internet to find the simplest definition.

---

6 Dr. Steven Gundry, "Welcome to Gundry MD", Gundry MD, Youtube, 17 June 2021, *https://www.youtube.com/channel/UC4ODXZL2r3XepieV0uoRjNA.*

7 Dr. Steven Gundry, "Dr. Gundry's Diet Evolution," The Ultimate Health Podcast, December 2017, *https://ultimatehealthpodcast.com/tag/dr-gundrys-diet-evolution/.*

> Mitochondria are known as the powerhouses of the cell. They are organelles that act like a digestive system, which takes in nutrients, breaks them down, and creates energy-rich molecules for the cell. The biochemical processes of the cell are known as cellular respiration.[8]

As I read that definition, I found another word I needed to look up: organelles. I turned back to the internet.

> An organelle is one small part of a cell that has a very specific function or job. The nucleus itself is an organelle.... Organelle is a diminutive of organ, from the idea that just as organs support the body, organelles support the individual cell.[9]

As I continued to listen and learn, it seemed that Dr. Gundry knew what he was talking about. I was especially fascinated when they started discussing aging. They discussed a study with animals where they took bacteria from a younger animal's gut and placed it in an older animal's gut of the same species. The bacteria made the older animal young again. That definitely got my attention.

I wondered how old Dr. Gundry was. According to my all-knowing internet, he was sixty-seven years old at the time that video was filmed. It was impressive that he had lost seventy pounds and looked younger than his age. He talked about a friend he'd recently had lunch with who was his same age but looked ten years older.

---

8 "Mitochondria — Turning On the Powerhouse," Rader's Biology4Kids.com, *http://www.biology4kids.com/files/cell_mito.html.*

9 "Organelle," Vocabulary.com, *https://www.vocabulary.com/dictionary/organelle.*

Then they started discussing fruits. Dr. Gundry said that plants have evolved, and they use a variety of strategies to protect themselves from animals and pests/bugs that want to eat them. Color is one of these defensive strategies. Unripe fruit, which is usually green, is hard to see for animals. Ripe fruit, which is usually red, yellow, or orange, signals sweetness to animals and to humans. Only animals that can see colors will eat fruits. When an animal eats a ripe fruit, the seed is fully cased. This means it can pass through the digestive tract to be deposited somewhere else to grow, something that is essential for a plant's propagation and survival. Eating unripe fruit makes animals—and humans—sick.

It used to be that humans would only eat fruit and vegetables when they were in season. Now, we eat fruit year-round without a second thought. But to do so, we pick them before they're ripe, load them up with chemicals that artificially change the color of the fruit, and ship them around the world.

We usually consider eating fruits and vegetables to be a healthy habit. However, Dr. Gundry argued that because of the unhealthy ways we harvest plants, they could actually be very detrimental to our health. This led to a term that I had not heard of before, called *The Plant Paradox.* It was a lot to comprehend, but my interest was piqued. I couldn't help but think of all the fruits and vegetables I had consumed during my daily juicing protocol.

Since I was a teenager and through most of my adult life, I have struggled with my gut. As a kid, there were times that I laid curled up in a ball because of the pain in my lower stomach. Bloating and gas were constant issues. In my late twenties, doctors diagnosed me with colitis. Back in those days, they used an inflexible camera and no type of sedation like they do today for colonoscopies.

I had one of my most embarrassing moments when my primary care doctor decided to invite a group of premedical students in to watch my colonoscopy. Back then, the doctor had you lay over a large wooden triangle naked so that your rear was sticking up in the air. I was lying face down, my knees and feet on the exam table with my bare bum stationed high on the peak of the triangle. I made the mistake of looking back. I could see that several of the students were cute, college-aged women, and they were staring right at the straight rod sticking out of my buttocks. Groaning, I just put my hands over my head while the doctor did the exam, taking his sweet time to slowly explain everything to his rapt students.

Because of the colitis and gut issues, I was sucking down Tums and a variety of other prescription medicines for indigestion. This was in addition to the NSAIDs I was pounding down daily. My colon issues worsened, and a doctor in Salt Lake City diagnosed me with Crohn's disease in 1992. Not one doctor during this whole agonizing time period ever discussed if there was anything that I might be eating that was causing my health issues.

You know, it's interesting: People who knew me at a surface level over all of these years would have thought I was the picture of health. I was very physically active. I looked fit. I was often tan due to my outdoor sports activities. I frequently traveled and stayed extremely busy with my demanding and prominent roles at work. Yet, writing this book has helped me realize how truly unhealthy I was—above and beyond the cancer. After reading this far into the book, you're probably thinking I was a mess! It's amazing how much we can ignore and compartmentalize the consequences of unhealthy behaviors in our lives.

Writing this book has finally put into black and white the horrible cycles that I was dealing with in regards to my volatile health. I would eat food and drink beverages that would cause burning at the top of my stomach. Then I would pound down the Tums. Later, I would get bloating in my stomach, which would lead to serious pain in my intestines, so I took a lot of Pepto Bismol to calm them down. Then I would have to go through the misery of expelling it all out through a colitis/Crohn's-diseased colon. I'll spare you additional details.

Dr. Gundry's podcast was making sense. I had had a real battle going on with my internal organs for most of my life, topped off with bladder cancer. I found that I had many questions, though. Was this restorative medicine practice that Dr. Gundry was touting real? Why would a world-renowned cardiologist who spent his career saving patients with heart disease change his practice to restorative medicine?

I found another podcast by Dr. Gundry and listened to it right then. He explained that he was tired of working with heart patients at the critical, life-saving surgery phase. He wanted to work with patients to prevent heart disease and heart failures. That made sense to me. He also explained how he had become a specialized research doctor because he had developed so many unique connections to top research facilities and associations throughout the world that were studying the cellular level of plants and humans.

The pain in my back as I sat for so long in my office chair reminded me of the harsh directive I was under to resist all NSAIDs, and I wondered what Dr. Gundry's opinion of them would be. I found an article online titled "Healthy Gut" by Nisha Gopalan. She quoted Dr. Gundry extensively, explaining that he believed finding the right bloat-free balance was as simple as eliminating some common drugs and foods that "wreck" (his strong choice of wording) your stomach. Then he said, "It's not what I tell you to eat, it's what I tell you *not* to eat."

I leaned into my screen to see what came next. Her article continued, "So what's on the banned list? Here's Dr. Gundry's Rx for living your best (digestive) life. 'Popping too many non-steroidal anti-inflammatory drugs (or NSAIDs), such as aspirin and ibuprofen, will damage your intestinal wall,' Dr. Gundry says."[10] I let out the breath I didn't realize I'd been holding. There it was. The number-one priority on his list to restore the gut and keep it healthy was to avoid all NSAIDs.

Over the past forty-seven years, I had seen more doctors than I could count. Until Dr. Khan, not one of them had ever even alluded to the negative effects of taking NSAIDs. They prescribed them for me. They encouraged me to take them, even. Not one concern had ever been raised about my over-the-counter pain medication addiction.

I was currently in the middle of my third hellish month of abstaining from NSAIDs. Between Dr. Kahn and Dr. Gundry, I was at a fork in the road. I now had two experts who had presented very strong cases for me to never take any form

---

10 Nisha Gopalan "3 Everyday Things That This M.D. Says Can Destroy Your Gut Health," Well + Good, 13 June 2017, *https://www.wellandgood.com/things-to-avoid-for-good-gut-health/.*

of those painkillers again. It all added up: I had all the gut problems they talked about. But I was still experiencing so much pain and swelling without those medicines. How would I ever be able to do it?

CHAPTER 10

HEALING MY LEAKY GUT

My health took a dramatic turn for the better in October of 2018. This wasn't a small improvement; I'm talking about a marked drop in overall body pain from head to toe. My stomach stopped bloating, and the pain in my lower stomach ceased completely. My bowels started functioning properly. Normally, I would go days without having a bowel movement, and when it would finally happen, it would be incredibly painful. What a shock it was to have a comfortable bowel movement on a daily basis. The burning in my feet from the peripheral neuropathy dropped 80% in pain level. My arthritis, which had been at a constant pain level somewhere between a four and an eight on a scale of ten, now caused little to no pain at all for days on end.

It was so weird to be walking around with no knee pain. I marveled at being able to grip tools and move chairs in our house without the swollen, sore feeling in my arthritic left hand. For an individual whose constant pain level had been in the five to eight range every day for years, to wake up one day with pain at only a two was unbelievably life-changing.

And I was experiencing this amazing change day in and day out without taking any NSAIDs at all for six months! This was miraculous to me. The gratitude I started feeling for Dr. Kahn and Dr. Gundry was indescribable.

Both of these doctors helped me to overcome my addiction to unhealthy pain medications, a major stepping stone in my journey toward full health. Dr. Gundry also helped me learn about another integral step: nutrition. From August 2018 through writing this book in 2021, Carla and I have learned just how much my nutrition—which I thought was top tier—was creating a negative inflammation cycle in my body. I learned that this cycle is called "leaky gut syndrome." The damage had started when I was a little kid and continued to haunt me as a grown adult until October of 2018.

What Is Leaky Gut?

Unless you live under a rock, you've probably at least heard the term "leaky gut" somewhere before. But do you know what that term really means? Before we continue, it's important to understand this concept. Please don't skip ahead, assuming "this doesn't apply to me." According to the experts, the chances are that it *does* apply to you, and probably to others you love as well. Having a leaky gut is actually a medical condition referred to as leaky gut syndrome. Doctors who specialize in leaky gut syndrome, like Dr. Gundry, assert that because of our modern lifestyle and environment, almost everyone is dealing with leaky gut.

Through much research and study, including Carla's in-depth functional nutrition training and interactions with Dr. Gundry and his staff, we've learned that most people aren't aware that they're dealing with a leaky gut because the symptoms go far beyond digestion. Symptoms can include digestive tract problems, such as gas, bloating, diarrhea, etc., but many people don't have digestive symptoms at all. Instead, what they have are one or more of the wide-ranging and seemingly unrelated other symptoms caused by a leaky gut. Here is a partial (emphasis on partial) list:

- Chronic fatigue and muscle pain
- Depression and anxiety
- Frequent sickness
- Inflammatory bowel disease
- Migraine headaches, brain fog, and memory loss
- Multiple food sensitivities or allergies
- Nutrition deficiencies
- Obesity and type 2 diabetes
- Psoriasis, eczema, and other skin conditions
- Seasonal allergies or asthma
- ADD or ADHD
- Insomnia or sleeplessness
- Food cravings and weight gain

When we treat these symptoms individually, it's as if we're putting a bandage on an open sore. To really get rid of these symptoms, we have to treat the root cause. If you have even one of these symptoms, chances are your problems stem from your gut. Leaky gut syndrome is also the main precursor to autoimmune diseases—things like Hashimoto's, lupus, rheumatoid arthritis, and celiac disease, to name a few.

Why does our gut have such an impact on our overall health? Because 60%–80% of our immune system sits in our gut. It's also where about 95% of our serotonin is produced, and serotonin is responsible for mood. The gut is essentially the gateway to health. As Dr. Amy Myers, another expert on leaky gut syndrome, puts it, "If your gut is healthy, chances are that you are in good health."[11] The opposite of this is equally true: If your gut is unhealthy, chances are that you're experiencing health problems. You just probably don't realize that the problems stem from your gut.

Here is a basic overview to help you better understand how the gut works. Your intestinal lining has two big jobs to do:

1. Absorb essential nutrients into your bloodstream
2. Keep dangerous toxins from entering your bloodstream

Because your intestinal lining has such important protective tasks to accomplish, it really is the first line of defense for your immune system. It is supposed to protect the bacteria in your gut microbiota and your overall gut health. The outside layer of the small intestine is bound by tight junctions. These junctions are meant to be semi-permeable so that the micronutrients we need to survive can pass through the intestinal wall and into the bloodstream. This is how we absorb food. Your gut provides the vital process that screens the food molecules passing through. The good stuff gets absorbed and provides us with energy and nutrients. The bad stuff keeps on going and eventually gets eliminated through your bowels. It's a beautiful system when it functions properly.

Leaky gut syndrome occurs when the tight junctions that keep your intestinal wall together become loose. When these

---

11 Amy Myers, MD, "9 Leaky Gut Symptoms & How to Heal," Amy Myers MD, 21 May 2021, *https://www.amymyersmd.com/article/signs-leaky-gut/.*

junctions are damaged, our gut barrier allows dangerous things, like undigested food particles, bad bacteria, or toxins, into our bloodstream. It may also mean that the good stuff—the nutrients our body wants and needs—are only partially absorbed. Our bodies react to these undigested food particles and toxins, marking them as threats and attacking them. Your body's immune response can appear in many different forms (see the list of symptoms mentioned above). This explains why a leaky gut leads to many autoimmune diseases because your body attacks itself. This may also be why you develop sensitivities or even allergies to certain foods; your gut has tagged it as a pathogen.[12]

One of the main side effects of leaky gut is fatigue. That's because fighting the harmful bacteria that get into your bloodstream is a big job! The longer it goes on, the more bad particles get released, and the harder your body has to fight. If you find that you are often tired and can't understand why, it may be a sign that you're experiencing leaky gut syndrome.

What Causes Leaky Gut?

Leaky gut is caused by a slew of external factors, many of which, quite frankly, are difficult to avoid. Much of our food today has been genetically modified, which greatly affects our gut. Toxins in our environment, such as pesticides and herbicides, affect our gut. Infections and inflammations, and the medications we take for them, affect our gut. Even stress affects our gut, causing the tight junctions of our intestinal walls to break apart.

---

12 Dr. Steven Gundry, MD, *The Plant Paradox*, (Harper Wave; 1st edition, 2017), pp. 71-92.

The more I studied and learned about leaky gut syndrome, the more I realized that what I put into my body mattered—really, *really* mattered. I thought I was a pretty healthy eater, but I discovered that what I considered healthy was likely damaging my gut. The experts seemed to agree that gluten was a major cause of leaky gut. That's because gluten is a lectin, and lectins are the bad guys. These small, dagger-like proteins break apart the tight junctions in our gut, and they aren't supposed to be in our bodies. Lectins are in a lot of foods we eat now because of things humans have done to alter food or soil or growing processes: foods like whole-grain wheat, eggplants, legumes, and tomatoes—all foods I had previously thought were good for me!

Although I thought I was a pretty healthy eater most of the time, I ate plenty of the foods on the lectin list. I also still had a weakness for bread; nothing compared to the crusty heaven of a fresh slice or a warm, home-baked roll. And another weakness still plagued me as well. I'd been fighting this vicious addiction since the days I'd consumed it by the bowlful as a kid—sugar. Although I'll save the sticky, sweet details for another chapter, sugar exacerbates every bad symptom associated with leaky gut.

I also learned that NSAIDs were another prevalent cause of leaky gut syndrome—yet another strike against them. I was a textbook case of someone in a vicious NSAID inflammation cycle: I'd have pain and inflammation somewhere in my body, so I'd take NSAIDs to lower the pain, which then damaged my gut lining and allowed bad bacteria into my bloodstream. This, in turn, caused increased inflammation in my body, so I'd take another round of NSAIDs. Over and over it went.

The things I was consuming were affecting my overall health in every way. They say you manage and protect your outside by managing what goes inside, and I'm a total believer. Once I started consuming the right things—and even more importantly, once I *stopped* consuming the wrong things, like sugar and bread and my daily dose of NSAIDs—I experienced a drastic improvement in health and a decrease in daily pain.

If Leaky Gut Is So Common, Why Isn't My Doctor Talking About It?

If it really is true that almost all of us have leaky gut issues, why isn't this on the forefront of every doctor's radar? Why had none of my doctors thought to discuss it with me as an underlying cause for my vast list of medical problems? The sad truth is that the medical community does not move very quickly. It actually takes an average of seventeen years for new research to make its way into clinical practice.[13] Seventeen years!

So why aren't physicians excited about this information? It's a pretty straightforward explanation for so many of the common ailments their patients are struggling with. Dr. Myers, who was trained as a conventional medical doctor before becoming a functional medicine physician, has an interesting explanation:

> Although gastroenterologists may recommend removing known gut irritants such as gluten for people with celiac disease or even a liquid diet for Crohn's disease, traditional medicine's approach

13 Zoë Slote Morris, Steven Wooding, and Jonathan Grant, "The answer is 17 years, what is the question: understanding time lags in translational research," Journal of the Royal Society of Medicine, December 2017, *https://www.ncbi.nlm.nih.gov/pmc/articles/PMC3241518/.*

> is generally treatment with harsh drugs including immunosuppressants and steroids.[14]

In other words, the medical world's go-to is prescribing to treat symptoms instead of treating or preventing the underlying cause. This is exactly what I'd been experiencing with all my doctors for decades. (If you are interested in additional information about the medical community and leaky gut syndrome, please see the note at the end of this chapter.)

Until I learned about all this in the fall of 2018, my diet and frequent consumption of pain medication had been the cause of so much pain and sickness in my life. By eliminating certain foods, including the majority of sucrose and fructose; giving up all NSAIDs (I have not taken any form of NSAID since May 2018); and utilizing proper health supplementation, I started healing my gut. The difference was dramatic and startling. The difference was wonderful. It felt like I had a whole new life.

Note:

Dr. Amy Myers is a well-known functional medicine physician who specializes in leaky gut syndrome. In her 2019 article titled, "Traditional Medicine and Leaky Gut," she explains:

> Leaky gut may be all over the media, yet it remains a controversial topic in the traditional medical community. Scientific evidence in controlled studies has shown that

14 Dr. Amy Myers, MD, "Is Leaky Gut a Medical Mystery?" Amy Myers MD, 6 September 2020, *https://www.amymyersmd.com/article/leaky-gut-medical-mystery/.*

> "increased intestinal permeability," or what we call leaky gut, plays a role in various gastrointestinal diseases, including Crohn's disease, celiac disease, and irritable bowel syndrome. However, one of the biggest debates in the medical community is whether or not leaky gut plays a role in other health issues.[15]

She goes on to explain groundbreaking research conducted by Dr. Alessio Fasano, an acclaimed Harvard researcher, which proved a protein called zonulin breaks open the tight junctions in the gut wall, which allows large, damaging particles to pass into our bloodstream. He also proved that wheat increases the production of zonulin and that there is a link between the opening of the gut wall, chronic inflammation, and autoimmunity.

Dr. Myers believes that once a drug has been developed that will treat the condition of leaky gut, its producer (big pharma) will then go to town marketing it. "I'm very confident the traditional medical community will be pushed to suddenly 'believe' in leaky gut and prescribe a costly medication to treat it, rather than address it through diet and lifestyle adjustments." This is the cycle that happens over and over again in the pharmaceutical and medical world. We keep patching holes through additional prescriptions.

---

15 Dr. Amy Myers, MD, "Is Leaky Gut a Medical Mystery?" Amy Myers MD, 6 September 2020, *https://www.amymyersmd.com/article/leaky-gut-medical-mystery/.*

CHAPTER 11

CONNECTING THE DOTS

I have lived through the following illnesses and major surgeries during my life:

1. Eczema most of the time, and so severe that both hands are covered completely.
2. Multiple strep infections that required antibiotics.
3. Multiple bronchitis infections that required antibiotics.
4. Multiple cases of pneumonia.
5. Diagnosed with colitis in my twenties.
6. Knee surgery in 1984.
7. Diagnosed with Crohn's disease in 1992.
8. Diagnosed with ADHD in 1999.
9. Diagnosed with peripheral neuropathy in 2000.
10. Knee surgery in 2003.
11. Shoulder surgery in 2006.
12. Groin surgery in 2006.
13. Foot surgery in 2007.
14. Swollen prostate and erectile dysfunction (ED) issues due to other health problems since about 2010.
15. Back surgery fusing S-1, L-5, and L-4 in 2014.

16. Bladder cancer surgery in 2015.
17. Second bladder cancer surgery in 2016.
18. Diagnosed with tinnitus in 2016.
19. Third bladder cancer surgery in 2016.
20. First round of chemotherapy for bladder cancer in 2016.
21. Second round of chemotherapy for bladder cancer in 2017.
22. Diagnosed with two forms of sleep apnea in 2017.
23. Diagnosed with melanoma cancer and had Mohs surgery in 2017.
24. Diagnosed with arthritis in my spine, right knee, and left hand in 2017.
25. Stem cell procedure in right knee in 2018.
26. Diagnosed with leaky gut syndrome in 2018.
27. Second back surgery in 2019.
28. Third back surgery taking out pre-existing hardware and fusing S-1, L-5, L-4, and L-3 in 2020.
29. Ongoing brain fog since initial back surgery in 2014.
30. Major dental surgery to remove four metal crowns, repair an existing root canal that had infection brewing in it, three old wisdom teeth that had infections, and removal of metal retainer on bottom front teeth that I had for thirty-two years in 2020.

I know that is quite the timeline of health issues! Putting it all together in a list is pretty humbling, and I hope my list is longer than yours. After thirty years of health issues, I was finally starting to connect the dots. Could it be that all of these issues had a common denominator?

One issue that plagued me for years was brain fog. This frustrating condition had begun with my first back surgery in October 2014 and worsened with each successive surgery.

My lack of memory and mental clarity was literally scaring me and driving me nuts. It was so bad I started asking myself, "Do I have the onset of dementia or Alzheimer's?" Most of our friends are dealing with parents who, like ours, are in their eighties and nineties. Many of them have their parents in memory care facilities or some type of assisted living because of senile dementia or Alzheimer's disease. A few years ago, my foster mom came to live with us, and she suffered from these conditions. The nine months she lived in our home were beyond challenging. My heart would hurt every time we had a bout with her dementia and hallucinations.

We'd been attributing my brain fog to the anesthesia I'd undergone, but as we researched, we realized it could also be a symptom of my leaky gut. The more I learned, the more I wanted to learn, and I was now reading and researching nonstop. Reading Dr. Gundry's book, *The Plant Paradox,* was a game-changer for me.

I decided I really wanted to find out if I had the Alzheimer's gene. I was driven to find out if Dr. Gundry could help me figure that out. I knew it was a long shot, but I took courage and contacted his medical office in Palm Springs, California. I asked the receptionist if he was still accepting new patients. To my total surprise, she said I could, in fact, work with Dr. Gundry, provided that I fill out some paperwork and provide blood samples for lab work.

"How hard can that be?" I asked myself. Carla's parents live in Palm Springs six months of every year, from November to April. We typically spend two weeks each year with them golfing, playing cards, eating out, going to their parties, and hanging out with their friends. We could easily make the time for a doctor's appointment while there.

I asked the receptionist when I could set up an appointment but was taken aback by her answer. "Dr. Gundry has hundreds of individuals wanting to be his patient," she drolly explained, as if she had rehearsed this for every one of them. "And he is only willing to meet with them based on certain criteria. First, you fill out all of the paperwork on your health history and other medical forms. Second, you are required to provide twenty-five vials of blood that will be split up between five laboratories. Third, your first visit will be with his physician assistant. Fourth, follow the recommended nutrition and supplementation program for one year. Fifth, repeat the paperwork and blood work again. Sixth, we will then schedule your first visit with Dr. Gundry."

I was totally flabbergasted. Was this for real? It never occurred to me that Dr. Gundry would need more than a year's worth of lab reports to really be able to work with a patient. I started to ask a question, but the receptionist was done with me. She'd already had to interrupt our conversation by placing me on hold multiple times to take other calls. She finally said, "You'll receive a packet in the mail in a couple of days and can begin the process." She hung up after I gave her my name and address. *Wow,* I thought. *This isn't a process; this is a long and laborious journey!*

I decided it was worth it, however. I thought of that long list of health challenges I'd had over the years, and the thought was sobering. It was especially sobering because, as I'd aged, my body's ability to heal itself had noticeably slowed. I'd first noticed this when I turned fifty. Then once I hit my sixties, it was a huge wake-up call to see how much slower—radically slower—my body was to heal, especially coming out of bladder cancer and chemotherapy. Plus, I wondered about my genetic medical history, which was mostly a mystery to me.

My mother was in her eighties, and she is a twenty-five-year breast cancer survivor. My biological father was adopted when he was a baby. I only met his adopted father a handful of times before he died when I was thirteen, but his adoptive parents' genetics had no bearing on my own. Over the years, I'd wondered so often about why I got sick so much. I'd tried to blame my frequent bouts of strep throat, bronchitis, and pneumonia on all the air travel I did for work, but I wished I knew if it was something genetic.

Once, in 1996, when I'd come home from a business trip yet again deathly sick with pneumonia, I went to my doctor of sixteen years and told him I was sick and tired of being sick. "What can I do to stop these constant illnesses?" I asked. His response was to write me a prescription for Prozac. I'm not proud of my reaction, but this really ticked me off. "Why in the world would a serious antidepressant help me overcome my sicknesses?" I demanded. He shrugged his shoulders and said it would help me sleep better at night.

You've probably heard of Prozac, but just in case you aren't familiar with it, Prozac is used to treat major depressive disorder, eating disorders, obsessive-compulsive disorder (OCD), panic disorder, and as part of the treatment for bipolar disorder. Here I was in his office for pneumonia, and he gave me two prescriptions: a serious antibiotic and Prozac. He instructed that if I didn't see improvement within twenty-four hours, I was to take myself to the hospital.

My mind was blown. Prozac? For pneumonia? There was a running joke in our community at the time about how many people were walking around like zombies because they were addicted to Prozac, the popular drug-of-the-moment. I had no desire to join the zombie club. I didn't mince words and told this doctor that both his advice and his Prozac prescription were ridiculous. I stomped out of his office without the Prozac and without any answers.

Over and over, I wondered, *Why am I so unlucky to be such a sickly person?* It was disconcerting to have so little information. What Dr. Gundry was offering totally intrigued me. Could I really use my blood work to better predict—and then prevent—any issues I could expect in my golden years? Armed with the information he said he could provide, could I proactively improve my health and create a better quality of life?

Between Dr. Khan and Dr. Gundry, I started connecting the dots as to the underlying causes of my painful and unhealthy life. Dr. Khan started me on the path to overcoming my daily NSAID use. Dr. Gundry started me on the journey to fixing my leaky gut. I looked forward with great anticipation to the upcoming lab work with Dr. Gundry. Although it was time-consuming and demanding, it was going to reveal so many things about my genetics that were dramatically affecting my health.

25 Vials

As soon as I got the paperwork from Gundry's office, I filled it out and mailed it back. Two weeks later, I received five small boxes from five different laboratories. Each box contained FedEx packaging, five vials to do a blood draw, and freezer packs to keep the specimens cold until the laboratories could process them. A few days later, I went to the Instacare they had suggested for doing the twenty-five-vial blood draw. Fortunately, the technicians there knew their stuff—no blown veins!—and it only took one hour to do the draws.

The hardest part was waiting for the results. Several weeks later, Dr. Gundry's office finally called and said they received all of my labs. The good news was that they could schedule my first appointment on December 5th, 2018, four weeks away, at 9 a.m. I enthusiastically accepted the date, and we planned our trip to Palm Springs. With Carla's parents living down there for the winter, we could visit them and continue my medical journey with Dr. Gundry.

The highly anticipated day finally arrived. The temperature in Palm Springs was a perfect seventy-two degrees. Thinking of the thirty-five-degree weather we'd left behind in Utah made it even more satisfying. Carla and I drove our white rental van to Dr. Gundry's office. It was somewhere near the airport, and there were lots of palm trees lining the streets.

Because of his prolific presence on the internet, his international reputation, and the many best-selling books he'd written, I'd been picturing a big, fancy office building with Dr. Gundry's picture and name in big letters on display. Boy, was I wrong! The GPS on my phone navigated us to an old, white, outdated office park. The parking lot was in the rear of the complex, and Dr. Gundry's office was toward the end of one of the buildings.

"Do you think we're in the right place?" I looked at Carla, who shrugged her shoulders. Where was the big building with his name in gold letters? As we walked up the cracked cement sidewalk between the worn buildings, I started having doubts.

Everything here looked old and tired. We approached the entrance, and there it was, a small plaque with Dr. Gundry's name on it. Carla and I looked at each other, like, "Well, I guess this is it!"

We walked into a tiny reception room with chairs lining three of the four walls. We approached the large opening in the fourth wall where the receptionist was sitting. She was in a small room, and we could see that two additional people were crammed in there, along with stacks and stacks of patient folders. There was a copier behind her, but it, too, had stacks of patient files on and around it, even on the floor. This was not at all what I was expecting from a world-renowned cardiac surgeon who had created a burgeoning restorative medicine practice.

"Hi, how can I help you?" the receptionist greeted us. I gave the receptionist my name, and she told me the physician assistant would be with us soon. Turning around, I peered at some framed plaques on the wall that showed off some of Dr. Gundry's accomplishments. There was a table in the corner with a bowl of nuts available for patients to eat as they waited. Another table hosted a stack of magazines titled *Our Health* by Dr. Gundry. I glanced around at the other patients—all several years older than I—sitting in the cheap waiting room chairs.

I grabbed a magazine and sat down, but before I could open it, I heard my name called. The PA had long, dark hair and dark-rimmed glasses, and her kind smile helped put me more at ease. After exchanging pleasantries, I leaned forward in my chair, anxious to get this meeting going. She pulled the first lab result out of the thick patient file on her lap and turned it around so we could read it.[16]

The first thing to catch my attention was all the elevated red scores on the first page. The words that stood out to me were, "Patient Acute Coronary Syndrome (ACS) Profile is elevated," and, lower down on the page, "This patient is at high risk and should be treated as such." I grimaced, realizing how much higher my chances are (3.51 times greater, specifically) that I would experience a heart attack than other men my age over a five-year period.

The second page of the report had way more red elevated scores than the green, normal range scores I was hoping to see. There were four red, two in the yellow (borderline) range, and two green scores. The first red elevated IL-16 measures immune formation and free radical damage. This is the signaling molecule that triggers the repair process; it is often associated with stress, obesity, and sleep apnea. This elevated score of 52.58 was very scary to me. At this point in our meeting, it was very difficult for me to stay positive.

What a wake-up call this was to see in bright Technicolor that I had an increased risk of heart attack! I glanced at Carla, wondering what she was thinking about it all. We still had four more lab reports to review, and I was hoping for some good news. The PA must've sensed my dismay and explained, "Just so you know, we use these reports to come up with a supplement augmentation plan in addition to a diet plan to solve the deficiencies that we find in these diagnostic reports. Let's move onto the next report from Salveo Diagnostics."

---

16 See list of laboratory reports in the appendix.

Looking over this report together, she pointed out on page one that my LDL-C (cholesterol) was high at 136 mg/dl and that we needed to work to lower it to under a hundred. This led to a short discussion on how important good fats like olive oil and avocados are to get these levels adjusted. Next, she pointed out that my triglycerides were mildly elevated, and to get them to optimal levels, I needed to lower my sugar and starch intake. I thought to myself, *That's easy for you to say since you might not be a sugar addict!*

On page two of this report, we finally got some really great news. For years I'd feared getting Alzheimer's or dementia as I aged. This was one of the main reasons I was sitting in this office. I followed along as the PA circled my ApoE Genotype marker, which was in the green, optimal range, and she explained that I was at no risk of developing Alzheimer's disease. I exhaled in relief. That was fantastic news and made me feel upbeat for a few minutes.

Page three showed that I have general inflammation in my body, which was caused by ingesting too much sugar. Next, it showed that I had the MTHFR gene. "What does that mean?" I asked her.

"It might look like a curse word at first glance, but it actually refers to a relatively common genetic mutation," the PA chuckled as she explained. "MTHFR stands for methylenetetrahydrofolate reductase. It's getting attention due to a genetic mutation that may lead to high levels of homocysteine in the blood and low levels of folate and other vitamins." The PA wrote on the report that I needed to take Methyl Folate and B12 supplements.

The first five lines on page five showed that my sugar addiction was mildly elevating my glucose and insulin. They showed that my sugars and proteins were in a mildly elevated range at two months out, and the fructosamine showed that my sugars were mildly elevated two weeks prior to the test.

Page seven showed my omega-3 index was mildly decreased, and she said I would need fish oil supplements. On page eight, under the heading "Gut Health Serum Assessment," it had both good and bad news. As I've shared before, I totally love bread and can eat lots of it at meals. The good news is that I don't have celiac disease. The bad news is that I am gluten intolerant. That explained all of the gut aches and pains that I had been dealing with on a daily basis.

This news came on the heels of my leaky gut research, so I'd already been trying to limit my bread intake. But knowing I was actually intolerant felt like a betrayal. *First, she tells me no sugar, and now I'm officially supposed to give up bread, too?* I felt the frustration building as the list of off-limit foods grew.

The only important news on page nine was that I needed to take a Ginkgo Biloba 120-mg supplement twice a day. On page ten, all of the markers looked good, and on page eleven, my total protein was high. The final news was that my complete blood count showed that I was not anemic.

The third report, "Vibrant Diagnostics," showed that the potential risk to develop celiac disease was unlikely. Everything else on the report looked good.

The Veridia Diagnostics report was all good news.

By the time we got to the fifth diagnostics report from True Health, I was just nodding at whatever the PA was saying. On pages one and two, I had three markers that showed intermediate risk. The PA wrote down the supplements that I would need to take to move those markers into the optimal range. It was a lot of information and felt so overwhelming. I was going to have to make some serious changes in my life.

At the conclusion of reviewing the reports, she presented us with a "Supplements Document" (see Appendix I) that she had been filling out during our discussion. She stated that most of them could be bought at Costco. I wondered if taking that many supplements would replace my daily meals and I could stop eating altogether, and I laughed out loud to myself. I was either going to laugh or cry! In the end, it was a lot to take in.

When we stood up, she said that we needed to make an appointment to see Dr. Gundry himself in a year. She stressed how important it was to follow the dietary guidelines and take the supplements. I would be required to get the blood work done again six to eight weeks before my appointment with him. With enthusiasm that I did not really feel, I agreed and thanked her for her time.

After setting the appointment and walking out of the office, I looked over at Carla to see if I could read anything on her face. She just seemed stoic. While opening the car door, I looked across the top of the car at her, but she was still unreadable. As we were getting our seat belts on, still nothing had been said between us.

I could no longer stand the silence and blurted out, "Well, how did you think that visit went?"

All stoicism suddenly gone, Carla answered, "That was amazing. I'm totally amazed at what they could do and all they could determine from your blood work! All of the recommendations they made about diet and supplementation were amazing."

Yeah, I thought to myself, *amazingly hard!*

All I could obsess about was that I had three-and-a-half times more chance of having a heart attack than other men my age, but Carla reminded me of the awesome news that I did not have the Alzheimer's gene. We were both very excited about that.

There was so much to discuss, and we decided to go straight to the Costco that was near the doctor's office to purchase the supplements. Carla, who was pretty much the picture of health, wanted to get started on some of the supplements, too, like the D3 and B12. At that moment, it felt like we had both joined together on an adventure. I was so thankful for her support in all of this.

Carla said that she wanted to read *The Plant Paradox* and learn for herself what the diet part of the protocol would be for the next year. This is what I love about her; when she gets on board, she is all-in. I also explained to her that Dr. Gundry had a cookbook that went along with *The Plant Paradox*. In our previous company, we had developed several cookbooks ourselves. We wanted to compare our current diet to his diet protocol.

Although I knew it wasn't going to be easy, and some of what I'd learned from all the lab results was difficult to hear, I really felt like today had provided many important answers.

We had connected the dots, and between these two doctors and all I'd learned, I was on the right path. The real work was about to start as I followed the diet, took all the supplements, and developed the discipline to be consistent. I wanted my appointment with Dr. Gundry the following year to be really memorable. I wanted to see dramatic improvement in all the negative markers. I couldn't wait to meet him in person.

CHAPTER 12

MEETING DR. GUNDRY: THE LEGENDARY PHYSICIAN OF RESTORATIVE MEDICINE

Unfortunately, the timing of my appointment with Dr. Gundry ended up overlapping with an extremely difficult recovery from yet another forced back surgery. Despite all I'd done to fix my back over the past years, the debilitating back pain had returned. It turned out the original surgery hadn't been done properly. After my first operation, the surgeon told me they should have gone up to the L3 vertebra, but since he hadn't requested insurance authorization for that, they simply hadn't done it. I was pretty furious when I found out.

In addition, every doctor I saw after that told me he'd actually done the wrong procedure, that it was an old-school surgery they don't do anymore. Lucky me. Long story short, on January 9th, 2020, I had the right surgery with the right doctor, who removed all my hardware and fused the proper vertebrae in the correct way.

I was in so much pain and discomfort from this major surgery that I told Carla I didn't want to do the labs and keep the appointment with Gundry. If I'm completely honest, however, my hesitation might have also been because I knew I hadn't been 100% faithful to the diet protocols I was supposed to be following over the past twelve months. I'd taken all my supplements faithfully; I hadn't missed a day. But bread and sugar remained my nemeses.

I'd cut out a substantial amount of sugar from my life, but many social functions I'd been attending over that year included a large table full of homemade goodies. Carla always made a sugar-free, gluten-free dessert, so there was something for me, but I couldn't keep myself from trying a bite or two of some of the other scrumptious-looking desserts.

An even bigger problem, however, was bread. Oh, how I loved bread! I had a neighbor who found out about my bread love affair who was a sourdough aficionado. She had a yeast starter that was over 100 years old and had been passed down through her family for generations. She brought us a warm, crusty loaf every week. Who could resist? Plus, I'd heard Dr. Oz quote Dr. Gundry as saying that sourdough bread was okay, so I figured I was fine. But deep inside, I worried all this would show up in my labs, despite how hard I'd worked to follow the many recommendations I'd received during my previous visit the year before.

Carla had other ideas. She'd had her own labs done and was scheduled to meet with Dr. Gundry's PA, and there was no way she was going to miss out on that. "David!" she exclaimed. "You've been so excited to meet *the* Dr. Gundry! And I really want to meet him, too. Plus, we've done all these supplements, we've been so faithful about taking them all, and I want to see if it makes a difference!" Needless to say, I kept my appointment.

On January 29th, Carla and I were back in his Palm Springs office. I was in a drug-induced haze on OxyCodone and five other medications from my surgery, but I really was highly motivated to meet Dr. Gundry in person. Luckily, Carla filled me in on all the details I couldn't remember later.

Carla had her appointment before mine with the same PA I'd met with last year. She was in pretty great shape; she'd always eaten healthily and didn't have the same struggles with gluten and sugar that I had. She'd also taken all the supplements with me since my last appointment.

Carla

I went to my appointment with Dr. Gundry's PA thinking I was doing pretty well. It's actually kind of hard to fill out all the intake forms required when you're healthy! I just kept marking, "No. No. No..." I did have a bit of knee joint pain after playing pickleball, and after seeing his chart about optimal stool size and texture (yep, it gets that up-close and personal!), I thought maybe mine could be a bit better, but that was it. But I was interested in seeing my lab results.

The PA had me add more fish oil for my joints, some milk thistle to help my liver metabolize the fish oil, and increased my Vitamin D. She also added a prebiotic to my regimen. Within four weeks, I had no joint pain. My bowel movements were perfect. Even better, though, was my energy. I had more energy than I'd had in a long time, and I had never considered myself to be a low-energy person. I had never complained about my sleep, but suddenly I was sleeping better than ever.

It was unbelievable. Things improved that I didn't even know needed improvement. I was amazed! All of this was such proof that even if your health is pretty good to begin with, a few small changes to your nutrition can equal truly meaningful, life-changing benefits.

David

Next up was my appointment with the man himself. We were led to a different office where Dr. Gundry was sitting behind his desk. Once again, I was surprised by his lack of pretension. Just as his office building lacked anything flashy or ostentatious, Dr. Gundry was just a regular guy. I'm not sure what I was expecting, but this world-renowned doctor/guru—the best-selling author who had been on Dr. Oz and has hundreds of thousands of followers, the doctor whose patients include the likes of Tony Robbins, Usher, and Randy Jackson—turned out to be a very down-to-earth, everyday, normal guy. He was also much smaller in person, tiny in his blue suit and big glasses on the other side of the desk.

"Hello!" he greeted and stood to shake our hands as we entered. He was very friendly and approachable, making us feel like we were old friends. He was also very old school; he didn't believe in technology, and the whole office operated on paper. I was itching to preach the convenience of going paperless and tell him how easily I could convert his whole practice but managed to contain the urge.

Dr. Gundry was very gracious as we introduced ourselves and made small talk with him. We said we'd read his books and watched many of his podcasts. I was enthused about how much better I was doing and how excited we were to see the lab reports; I just knew I was going to be 100% better. To myself, I thought, *We were good 90% of the time with diet and 100% with supplementation. Will it be good enough to improve my potential heart disease numbers? I was definitely nervous. Would he be able to tell all the times I cheated with sugary snacks and sourdough bread?*

Fidgeting with his pile of papers and notes (doesn't he know this could be so much easier on a laptop?), Dr. Gundry pulled out my PULS Cardiac Test Results for both 2018 and 2019 (see Appendix I). He was very fatherly and kind as he showed me my results, but all I could see was my elevated score jumping off the page at me from the very end of the bright-red, dangerous side of the scale.

I had to squint to make sure I was reading these shocking scores correctly. My PULS score of 15.88% put me in the "absolute risk" category and was double the number at the highest end of the chart. The expected score for someone my age and gender was 3.11%. My numbers meant I had 5.11 times the chance of other men my age of experiencing a heart attack in the next five years.

Even in my drug-induced stupor, loud warning bells were going off in my brain. How could this possibly be? Perhaps I was remembering last year's scores incorrectly? I asked Dr. Gundry if he could show us the 2018 report. "Sure," he said, shuffling through the papers and pulling it out. I was horrified to see the previous year showed my score was 10.38%.

Somehow after working hard for over twelve months, my risk of heart attack had actually increased. How could this be? I felt sick to my stomach, and I knew it wasn't from the medications I was taking. Both Carla and Dr. Gundry could tell I was upset and discouraged. As calmly as I could, I turned to Dr. Gundry. "What happened? I took all the recommended supplements. I was 90% compliant on the diet." I put my hands out and shrugged, like, "Come on, man!"

Dr. Gundry looked down at the reports, shuffled some papers, and smiled as he looked up at me. "David," he said, his voice warm and kind, "there is a lot of improvement on almost all of your metrics. You moved so many markers. What you've been doing is working! Your IL-16 is the only one highly elevated. But you're right—this one definitely matters. We need to get this number down. This elevated index is caused by lectins." He took his pen and noted this by the elevated red portion of the graph. He had an impressive ability to write upside-down from his side of the desk.

I knew from reading his books and listening to his podcasts that lectins were troublemakers. Lectins are large proteins found in plants and animals, and they wreak havoc on your digestive system. The one lectin you've probably heard of is the infamous gluten, but there are many others that are even more problematic. These sticky proteins interrupt messaging between our cells, causing toxic and inflammatory reactions. They are, essentially, edible enemies that are found in the vast majority of the American diet today, including bread.

I was leaning forward and listening so intensely my back started to hurt. Feeling defeated, I eased back into my chair as he asked, "Did you remove bread completely from your diet?"

I glanced at Carla and then sheepishly looked back at him. "We have done a great job, with one exception. We followed your advice, and now we only eat sourdough bread."

He looked taken aback. "Where did you get that notion from? I advised that sourdough was okay?"

"Well, yeah. We watched the clip on YouTube of you on *The Dr. Oz Show*, and you said sourdough bread was safe." My confidence faltered. "In fact, Dr. Oz said that according to you, it's the safest bread choice, better than both white and whole-grain, right?"

This made Dr. Gundry tilt back in his office chair. He tucked his chin into his neck and contemplated how to respond. Then he looked back at us. "It was important to Dr. Oz to have some type of bread that his audience could eat. Sourdough is suitable for many gluten-sensitive individuals; with fast-rising yeast, the bacteria don't have time to do any pre-digesting. But sourdough bread still has lectins in it, as well as some gluten. Obviously, your system is particularly sensitive to both. Going forward, you must stop eating all gluten and cut out anything, including vegetables, that has lectins in it."

I leaned forward again and put my elbows on his desk, resting my head on my hands. I decided it was time to come clean. "Our good friend Becky has a yeast start that goes back over 100 years. She makes the most amazing sourdough bread and gives us a big loaf every week. It makes the best toast.

You just have never had anything better than that bread with some homemade raspberry jam smeared on it. It might be my favorite part of every day, that piece of toast!"

After I wrapped up my sourdough testimonial, Dr. Gundry started to laugh. "Not only are you going to cut out that bread, but that raspberry jam is filled with sugar! You've got to make sure your sugar intake is minimal."

My heart sank. Could I really give up my beloved bread and jam? I glanced again at the page with the bright-red, high-risk results and swallowed. With a chagrined look at Dr. Gundry, I said, "Yes, sir," only half-joking. Then I had another thought. "Is there any chance that the back surgery I had last February, and the complications I've battled from that since May, could be spiking these numbers? I really have been suffering from it immensely, and the last year was so stressful… I'm hopeful that this recent surgery will be successful and lower my pain and stress, but… could that be affecting these numbers?"

"Sorry," he countered. "The surgeries have little bearing on the IL-16. You must modify your diet as I've suggested."

Well, I thought to myself, *it was worth a shot.*

Although I was still fixating on these negative numbers, Dr. Gundry started to review the other lab reports with me. We reviewed the information from Salveo Diagnostics next. My year-over-year lipids had improved slightly. The inflammation and oxidative stress metrics had improved. I needed to increase my Vitamin D from 10,000 to 15,000 IUs daily, but my Vitamin B12 was right in line.

Eleven of the diabetes– and insulin-resistant numbers were optimal, with only two that needed some work. The cardiac stress was in the optimal range. On the RBS Fatty Acid Profile, eleven of the twelve indicators were optimal. My Omega-3 index was mildly decreased, so Dr. Gundry increased my fish oil supplementation from two to four capsules daily.

The celiac disease indices were optimal, and the thyroid workup was optimal with year-over-year improvement. The hormonal health, bone health, electrolytes, kidney function, liver assessment, proteins, iron studies, and complete blood counts were all optimal as well. My cardiometabolic report from Quest lab looked good, too. At this point, I was feeling pretty good about myself, and Dr. Gundry was nodding positively as we reviewed each lab. It seemed my hard work over the past year was paying off.

Next, he pulled out the Supplements Page from my appointment the year before, crossed out the 2018 date, and wrote 1/29/2020 on it instead. He went through and marked any of the dosage changes we'd discussed, all with that impressive upside-down handwriting.

Once we'd finished reviewing the lab results, Dr. Gundry returned to a previous topic. "Let's talk more about that sugar intake issue," he said. He then spent the next forty-five minutes simply educating us about sugar. It was obvious he truly cared that we understood and was willing to take whatever time necessary to teach us the truth about this harmful substance. "Did you know that eating any kind of sugar can potentially reduce your body's defenses by 70% for up to six hours after eating it?" He looked pointedly at me. "Sugar in raspberry jam is an easy one to identify and remove from your diet. There is sugar hiding in plenty of other places that are much sneakier. Here, let me show you."

He pulled a box of crackers down from a shelf that was lined with various packaged foods. "Look at that label," he said, handing the box to us. "According to the label, there is zero sugar per serving, right?" We nodded, noting that the label said zero grams of sugar. "Manufacturers have manipulated the system to hide the sugar content," he explained. "That number just refers to added sugar. Here's how I want you to read nutrition labels. Take a look at the total carbohydrates." We looked and saw it said thirteen grams. "Okay, that's the total number of sugar molecules in grams. Then you take the fiber and subtract that number from the carbohydrates, and that gives you the actual grams of sugar per serving. So how much sugar is in each serving of those crackers?"

We did the math, subtracting the one gram of fiber from thirteen, and answered, "Twelve grams."

"Grams don't mean much to most of us, so here is an easy tip: There's four grams of sugar in each teaspoon. So, divide that twelve by four; there's about three teaspoons of sugar in a serving of crackers. That's three teaspoons of sugar in every five crackers you eat."

We were shocked. Who knew we had to worry about sugar in crackers?

"One piece of whole wheat bread has the equivalent of four teaspoons of sugar in it," he continued. "One bagel has eight or nine teaspoons of sugar. There's about twelve teaspoons of sugar in a can of soda. So a bagel has almost the same amount of sugar as a can of non-diet, sugary soda, and it doesn't even taste sweet! A bagel is actually higher on the glycemic index than sugar soda, which means one plain bagel will spike your blood sugar level faster than a can of soda does."

He continued to pull other food items off the shelf and reviewed the labels with us. One of the worst offenders is cereal. We don't eat much of that, luckily, but my very favorite to splurge on with my grandkids is Cinnamon Toast Crunch. By looking at the label, you'd think it had twelve grams of sugar. Nope, that's just the added sugar. The wheat has sugar, too. So you take the thirty-three total carbs from one serving and subtract the two grams of fiber, which equals thirty-one grams. Divide that by four (the teaspoons in each gram), and you realize that for each cup of cereal you eat, you're consuming eight teaspoons of sugar. No more Cinnamon Toast Crunch for me ever again!

Our minds were pretty blown. We had no idea how fraudulent and misleading food labels were. Millions of people, including us, have been led astray by the food industry, and as a result, we are a nation of addicts. Sugar in any form—whether it be fructose, glucose, starch, honey, maple syrup, or the all-natural cane sugar itself—is highly addictive.

In fact, when rats or mice who have been previously addicted to heroin or cocaine are given a choice between those drugs or sugar water, they will go for the sugar every time. Science tells us why: Sugar hits the same pleasure centers in the brain that heroin and cocaine hit, but sugar hits even harder.[17] It's no wonder we love sugar! And that it's so hard for us to give it

17 Magalie Lenoir, et al. "Intense Sweetness Surpasses Cocaine Reward," US National Library of Medicine and National Institutes of Health, August 2007, *https://www.ncbi.nlm.nih.gov/pmc/articles/PMC1931610/.*

up. I had known I was a sugar addict for a while now, but what I didn't realize was how much of that wasn't my fault.

We thanked Dr. Gundry profusely and promised him that next year our panels would reflect our commitment to our health. Then we drove straight from our appointment to Costco, just like the year before, but this time we spent our time there reading labels. We thought we'd been eating pretty healthy, but now that we were reading food labels differently, we realized we had to make even more changes.

I was fixated on that one bad number again and the fact that my chances for a heart attack were so high. I knew now I'd been rationalizing so I could keep enjoying that delicious sourdough bread, but I had to change. I had to be 100% all-in. It was time to stop living to eat... and time to start eating to live.

Note: We did not record these sessions with Dr. Gundry. We are sharing these memories as accurately as we can recall and based on all notes, appointment paperwork, etc.

CHAPTER 13

THE LAST DOT REVEALED: VISCERAL FAT

Five months had passed since our meeting with Dr. Gundry. My back was healing well, and—hallelujah!—I finally had no pain in my lower spine. What a relief! My overall health was improving. I met with my neurologist and explained my goal of getting off all medications. I asked if I could wean off the prescription medication I was currently taking for foot pain. He agreed, and we formulated a plan to step dosage down over the next month. After that, I'd just have two prescription medicines left—a vast improvement for me.

I'd come so far in my quest for optimal health: I'd learned about the far-reaching effects of proper nutrition and supplementation and the strong brain-gut connection. I had overcome a pretty extreme addiction to NSAIDs and other pain relievers that were wreaking havoc on my system. I'd figured out the sleep connection and was now consistently getting quality, reparative sleep each night. I knew my system was particularly sensitive to those dangerous lectins, and I was diligently avoiding all gluten. I was trying to calculate carbs and sugar in the proper way, now that Dr. Gundry had taught me how to read those misleading and tricky food labels. But, even with all this, there was still one important puzzle piece missing.

A couple of years ago, I had overheard Carla talking to our daughter, Whitney. They were discussing a Dexa Body Scan that Whitney had done. She'd discovered a company that uses a BodySpec DXA scanner (also known as Dexa Scan) that gives an accurate and specific body readout, including lean muscle mass, fat mass, bone density, and body symmetry. This is done using a GE advanced scanner with very weak x-ray beams.

Carla's mom has osteopenia, a form of bone loss that often precedes osteoporosis, so she was immediately interested in learning more about her bone mineral content. I perked up, too, interested in improving my overall health. Carla had already made an appointment. Not one to be left out, I called and got scheduled for an appointment right after hers. We had our first body scans done in June of 2018.

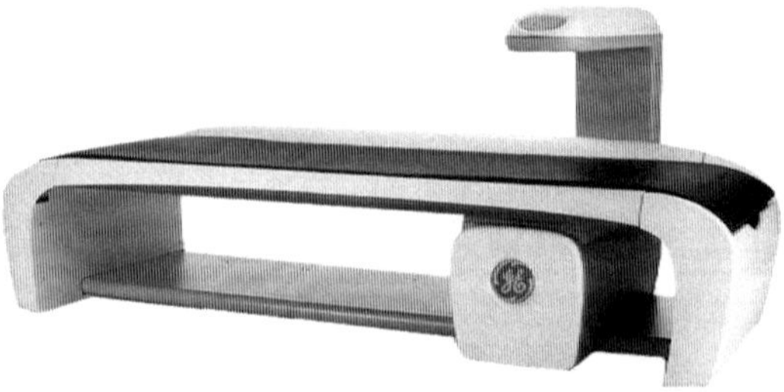

The BodySpec DXA Scanner

Getting a body scan is easy, painless, and relatively fast. All you have to do is lie down on the table and listen to the hum of the scanner as it moves up your body. Then you meet with the technician, who will review the detailed information with you in layman's terms. Basically, your first scan gives you a baseline of where you are, and from there, you can set realistic and achievable goals. Then you can use subsequent scans to see if your fat and lean muscle percentages have changed in positive or negative directions.

They reviewed Carla's results first. It was fascinatingly detailed, showing percentages by body part, even comparing right and left, front and back. Carla, who is lean and fit and whom most would consider to be an active, even athletic, woman, had 35% body fat. That surprised us both. The healthy range of body fat for men is typically defined as 18%–24%, while the healthy range for women is 25%–31%.[18]

It was interesting to see that her right arm and leg both had considerably more muscle than her left, but it made sense when we thought about the types of sports she played. She was right-side-dominant in tennis, pickleball, and golf. Years ago, when she was training with our son Skyler, he had warned her that she was really right-side dominant and should probably do additional strength training with her left. The scan had proved him right.

Her primary concern, however, and the main reason for getting the scan, was to see her bone density or bone mineral content. She was pleased to see that her results in this area were very

---

18 "Tools and Calculators," American Council on Exercise, *https://www.acefitness.org/education-and-resources/lifestyle/tools-calculators/percent-body-fat-calculator/.*

good for her age. "This is good," Carla said, turning to me. "We're doing this so we can see what effects real change, right? This is really going to show us if what we're doing is working."

We then turned to my results. I had a total body fat index of 26.5%, which is above the normal range of 18%–24% for my age (based on the American Council for Exercise's recommendations). *How annoying for an amateur athlete!* I immediately thought to myself. The technician continued her explanation, and the report revealed that thirty-four pounds of fat resided in my trunk. That explained the paunch and love handles that never seemed to completely go away, no matter how hard I worked on reducing them.

We left with our reports in hand and had a robust conversation in the car while driving home. We discussed working out hard for the rest of the summer and eating right, then getting a scan again three months later. Carla was highly motivated to reverse her fat tissue and increase her lean muscle tissue while evening out her left and right muscle mass. I wanted to chip away at those pounds of fat on my trunk. Once you see your body composition in color, it really motivates you to do something about it! We wanted to see a difference at the next scan.

The bad news for me was that I jacked up my back golfing with friends, which ultimately resulted in another back surgery a few months later. Frustratingly, this injury kept me from being able to work out seriously. I was able to ride my road bike on the trail behind our house several times a week, but that was about it. We returned for our second scans in September. Carla saw progress on all of her goals. I found I had lost two pounds of fat tissue and gained one pound of muscle, the net effect being that I had lost one pound in three months. The same technician we saw before was encouraging about the improvement.

Meanwhile, life went on. During the two years that followed, I learned about leaky gut syndrome, had my appointments with Dr. Kahn and Dr. Gundry, and had two more painful back surgeries. I'd all but forgotten about the body scanning until I overheard my wife and daughter talking about Carla going to get another scan. Since my appointment with Dr. Gundry, I'd been trying (and failing) not to obsess about the fact that I had five times the normal risk of heart attack and decided I wanted to get another scan as well.

In June 2020, I had my third body scan. The same friendly technician administered the scan, and then we discussed the results. This time, however, there was a new column of information on the report. "We got a software upgrade!" the tech shared enthusiastically. "Now, we can get a clear picture of your visceral fat." She turned to the third page of my report and pointed out that I had 5.29 pounds of Visceral Adipose Tissue (VAT).

"Is that a bad number?" I asked, not knowing what visceral fat meant.

"Well, a healthy individual should have less than one pound of VAT."

One pound or less? And I had over five? That was rattling, to say the least. As she was speaking, I was scanning the verbiage at the top of the page and saw that VAT is associated with metabolic diseases. I asked her, "Are heart disease and type 2 diabetes metabolic diseases?"

With her sweetest voice, she said, "Yes, they are, Mr. Meine."

At this point, my heart stopped for a beat. I asked myself, "Could visceral fat be the reason that I have a five-times greater chance of having a heart attack than men my same age?" As it turned out, I was exactly right.

Silent but Deadly: Visceral Adipose Tissue (VAT)

We all know that excess body fat isn't good for us, but there is a type of fat that is significantly worse than others. The culprit is visceral fat, and although it makes up only a small proportion of body fat, it plays a key role in some pretty troublesome health problems. Visceral fat—or intra-abdominal fat—can't be pinched by your fingers. It wraps around your abdominal organs, such as the liver and intestines deep inside your body. You can't feel it or see it, except perhaps through a growing waist size. Visceral fat leads to serious medical issues, including heart disease, Alzheimer's, type 2 diabetes, stroke, and high cholesterol.

The trouble with visceral fat cells is that they are biologically active. They secrete hormones and other molecules that mess with other tissues. Visceral fat produces proteins called cytokines, which trigger inflammation that leads to high blood pressure and other chronic conditions such as those listed above. It also produces a protein that increases insulin resistance. (For some eye-opening stats on specific ways visceral fat is implicated, see the notes at the end of this chapter.)

Where you gain fat depends on a handful of things, including your genes, hormones, age, gender, birth weight (believe it or not, smaller babies add belly fat more readily later in life), and whether you've had children or not. Things like birth weight and menopause are out of your control, but there are things we can do to minimize visceral fat. It actually responds more efficiently to diet and exercise than the subcutaneous fat on our hips and thighs does. You don't even have to do anything too crazy. A mere thirty minutes of moderate-intensity activity a day makes a big difference.

I finally understood why, despite all the healthy changes I had made, I still had such a high chance of heart attack. I had struggled so much with my "heart disease revelation" since my meeting with Dr. Gundry five months ago. I couldn't understand how to get those numbers down. Part of my dilemma was that I was also recovering from yet another back surgery, and other than physical therapy, I hadn't been able to really focus on optimal health. Then the COVID-19 pandemic hit, keeping me stuck at home and forcing my life to become even more inactive. But now, I knew I had to get those internal, visceral fat pounds down! It could be life or death for me!

Seeing those VAT numbers staring back at me gave me a tremendous motivator—my WHY—to improve my health. It gave me a specific target. Could I really focus on losing visceral fat? I began formulating a plan about how to go about losing VAT as the ideas pulsed through my mind. I was highly motivated to see those numbers decrease in my next scan three months from now.

Here is the plan I came up with to lose the visceral fat around my organs:

1. Five days a week of aerobic training. Multiple studies confirm that cardio will help you lose this fat faster than dieting. My cardio of choice is riding my road bike. I have lots of hills that require effort and move my heart rate above 149 beats per minute. Typically, on the bike ride, I will average 125 bpm.
2. No sugary snacks.
3. I'd stay committed to my plan to eliminate all breads! Since I am gluten intolerant, this is a must.
4. 15 minutes a day of guided mindful meditation.
5. Eating smaller portions. This is really difficult and is a habit that I want to develop for the rest of my life.

Three Months Later

In September, I had another body scan. In just three months, I'd lost 1.5 pounds of visceral fat. I dropped eight pounds of subcutaneous fat and gained ten pounds of muscle. I had worked hard and followed my plan, and my strategies were obviously working! It felt like such a victory. I was now even more motivated and committed to seeing the results of my next scan in six months. I celebrated with a sunset bike ride, feeling on top of the world.

After all these years, after all the sleuthing and researching and doctors and tests and surgeries, at last, I felt I had the final puzzle piece in place. Although achieving and maintaining optimal health is an ongoing journey that requires ongoing effort, I truly felt I'd finally connected all the dots on my way to optimal health. I'd worked hard to figure it out, and I intend to work just as hard every day for as long as I have left because, as the famous anthropologist Ashley Montagu said, "The idea is to die young as late as possible."[19]

Carla

I've been doing these body scans for a couple of years now. I love how specific the readouts are and find it really motivational. The number-one reason I get the scans is to see how my bone density is doing. Knowing that osteoporosis is potentially in my genetic makeup, I plan to work hard to keep my bones healthy. Research says there are three things I can do to impact my bone mineral content: exercise, take vitamin D, and take calcium supplements. I've been doing all three very intentionally for my bone health, and the body scan tells me if it's working.

I hadn't been too worried about my lean/fat ratios, but when I saw the numbers on the page, I thought, *Oh my gosh! I've gotta do something about that!* I was already pretty physically active, but I upped my game just a little bit to see if I could get those numbers to move at the next scan in two months.

So, in addition to the occasional pickleball game, and the cycling ride I sometimes do, I joined a walking group, walking with neighborhood friends a few days a week. I also added twenty minutes of medium-intensity weightlifting three times a week. But it wasn't anything crazy. Ten years ago, I was using thirty-five and forty-pound weights to work out. But now, I use

19 "Ashley Montagu Quotes and Sayings - Page 1," inspiringquotes.us, *https://www.inspiringquotes.us/author/4575-ashley-montagu.*

a twelve-pound dumbbell in each hand as I do my squats and lunges. Also, because I am so right-side dominant, I increased my reps by 50% on my left side. That means if I did ten bicep curls with both arms, I would do an extra five with just my left. I wanted to see if I could start to even my arms and legs out.

I also cracked down on my diet. I was already eating fairly clean, but I became more vigilant in taking my supplements and drinking my green drinks. The biggest change, however, was cutting out sugar. I wouldn't eat sugar in front of David—that would've been plain mean—but I was still sneaking in my little sugar fixes! It wasn't much, but I'd have a little treat here or there. I knew sugar affected David negatively, but I'd been telling myself that it wasn't affecting me. I could still have my little sugar treats!

Perhaps it wasn't affecting me much on the outside, but sugar is a time bomb waiting to go off for my insides. So the main change I made was that I really tried to stay away from sugar in the way that Dr. Gundry taught us, by calculating accurate grams on all food labels. Then I was consistent. Consistency was key.

When I went back two months later, I was completely blown away by the results. Here I was at sixty-two years old, and in just eight weeks, I saw those numbers really move. In two months, I reduced my overall body fat by 4%. I lost six pounds of fat and gained four pounds of muscle. I reduced the percentage of fat in my trunk. I was very pleased to see that my right and left sides were almost equal in muscle mass now, after just eight weeks of moderate-intensity workouts. And my bone mineral content had improved. I was relieved to see that my visceral fat, or VAT, was under one pound, the recommended amount. But

I was shocked and ecstatic to see how much a sixty-two-year-old woman could affect all those other areas just by putting in a little extra effort and by doing it consistently.

We recently returned from a family trip with all of our kids and grandkids to Island Park. These gatherings can be quite challenging when it comes to healthy eating. There are treats and sugary snacks, and yummy, carb-loaded meals everywhere. But for every grandkid-friendly meal, we also offered a healthy alternative, and I was so impressed as David ate his salads and gluten-free meals. In the past, he would've caved for sure, giving in to some dessert here and a snack there. But this time, he did so well. He was amazing! He'd had his body scan before we left and now knew about those ominous extra pounds of visceral fat. He just looked at me and said, "I'm getting rid of this visceral fat. I am not having a heart attack after all this work!" His "why" was sitting all around him—he wants to be around for those grandkids for a long time to come!

Additional Visceral Fat Information

Visceral fat is implicated in many chronic conditions. Here are a few you might want to know about:

- **Cardiovascular disease:** Waist size directly affects the risk of heart disease. Studies show that people with the biggest waist (in relation to their hip size) have more than double the risk of developing heart disease. This remained true even when adjusting for other factors, such as blood pressure, smoking, cholesterol, etc. Every two inches of additional waist size raised the risk for cardiovascular disease by 10%.

- **Dementia:** Research shows that people in their early forties with the highest levels of abdominal fat, compared with those with the least amount of abdominal fat at the same age, were nearly three times more likely to develop dementia, including Alzheimer's disease, later in life.
- **Colorectal cancer:** Research also shows that people with the most visceral fat have three times the risk of developing precancerous polyps than those with the least visceral fat.
- **Breast cancer:** Several studies found that premenopausal women who carried extra weight around their abdomen were at greater risk for breast cancer.
- **Asthma:** A large study found that women with high levels of visceral fat were 37% more likely to develop asthma, even if their overall weight was normal. Researchers believe belly fat raises the risk of asthma due to its inflammatory effects throughout the body, including your airways.

Additional information about how visceral fat affects these conditions can be found at https://www.health.harvard.edu/staying-healthy/taking-aim-at-belly-fat.

Note: In Appendix I, you can see the Dexa Body Scan report that includes the VAT numbers. You can see the hardware from my two fusion surgeries—they stand out in dark black in the picture. You can even see, through the shape of my spine, the mild scoliosis I have that has gotten worse with the fusions.

CHAPTER 14

MY ONGOING BATTLE WITH MY GREATEST NEMESIS: SUGAR

We'd done it. We'd put in the work, and through much research, education, doctor visits, treatments, and diet and lifestyle changes, Carla and I believed we had the answers to living our best, healthiest lives. But that didn't mean there weren't ongoing challenges and daily temptations to face. My WHY is strong, but the pull of one of my greatest nemeses—sugar—is pretty strong, too. Perhaps some of you can relate.

Sugar in the form of ice cream is a particular problem. When I walk past a Baskin Robbins or Cold Stone Creamery, it's like the logical, rational part of my brain is instantaneously hijacked! Suddenly, I can't think of anything else; that ice cream calls to me, and I can't see beyond the sweet, creamy scoops! In Greek mythology, a siren is a half-bird, half-woman creature who lures sailors to their destruction by the sweetness of their song. Ice cream is my personal siren. All my commitment to nutrition and health goals suddenly seems a lot less important once my nose sniffs out a freshly baked waffle cone. I'll take all the scoops, please!

Although it may be my favorite, ice cream is not my only sugar vice. Sugar and I go way back. From the time I was a little kid, up until about seven years ago, I drank soda like crazy. My beverage of choice was an ice-cold Coca-Cola. I worked at a grocery store as a teenager, and it was not uncommon for me to drink two or three cans of Coke a day. It didn't take many drinks until I acquired a taste for and really craved those sugary, carbonated beverages. I had no idea that one can has 39 grams of sugar and 140 calories!

My sugar addiction included Hostess treats and candy bars (especially Snickers), but donuts and pastries and especially homemade baked goods remain a fierce sugar temptation today. Chocolate chip cookies with macadamia nuts are absolute kryptonite to my willpower. I'm going into a sugar coma just writing about it!

For many years, I had a routine each night that included doing multiple rounds through my kitchen—basically a sugar scavenger hunt. I'd start with the refrigerator and freezer, then move on to the cupboards where I knew we kept processed foods. Then I'd scour the countertops and sift through the pantry. Some nights I'd exercise a bit of self-discipline, but most of the time, if I found something I liked, I'd gobble it down as a bedtime snack.

You're probably picturing me as a roly-poly chubbers with three chins wearing high-waisted, big-man pants after that long and descriptive (although by no means complete!) sugar-addiction confession. But here's the thing—I'd never been a fat guy. I thought I could get away with eating whatever I wanted because I was a fit guy!

Remember, when I met Carla, my profile picture was of me crossing the finish line at a recent triathlon. That wasn't a bait-and-switch attempt; I really was that guy. While we were dating and during the first years of our marriage, I was training for high-endurance events like the Ironman race. I spent at least twenty-five hours a week intensely swimming, biking, and running. I looked good, and I felt good! I knew I was supposed to carb load for this kind of training and competing, and because of my extreme training schedule, I thought I could just choose whatever carbs I wanted. When Carla met me, I was eating a bowl of ice cream every single night. I remember it blew her away. I was following a competitive triathlete's social media, and she said she always ate a whole pan of brownies the night before a race. I interpreted that to mean I could eat what I wanted, carte blanche.

Then, Carla decided to join me in my training and racing. It was awesome doing it together, and we worked out and trained hard. Before we were married, Carla was a pretty healthy eater. I'm sad to say that instead of being influenced for good by her, I brought her over to the dark side. We'd carb load together before a race by eating pasta and cookies and all the junk we wanted. And we were fit, and we did well, and we looked good (well, I can certainly vouch that Carla looked darn good!), but we had no idea the damage we were causing on the inside with all the crap we were putting in our bodies.

Who knows how much better we could've done in those races had we made better choices? If we'd fueled our bodies with starchy vegetables and plenty of healthy, leafy greens, would we have performed better? More importantly, would I have avoided some of the health pitfalls that—despite being fit and strong and looking healthy—I found myself facing over the past decade? We get so caught up in thinking that being healthy is about looking a certain way or maintaining a certain weight. I'm living proof that this is a dangerous fallacy.

When we started our fitness company, I began researching sugar. I was pretty staggered by what I learned, and in 2013 I first attempted to overcome my sugar addiction. I wrote and published a book called, *Think: Use Your Mind to Shrink Your Waistline.* I found a study from 2010 that stated the average American consumed 130 pounds of sugar a year. In 1805, the average American consumed five pounds of sugar per year.[20] After considering what I had been eating, I realized I might be an outlier, eating even more than the 100+ pounds the average Joe was eating. I sure hope that you eat way less sugar than I did!

I'd like to quote part of a chapter about sugar from my previous book:

> Sugar is responsible for triggering both an adrenal response, (the "rush") and the release of serotonin, (the "ahhh"). When these excited and happy feelings subside, we want to experience them again. And each time, we have to eat or drink a little more sugar to get

---

20 "How Much Sugar Do You Eat? You May Be Surprised!," Health Promotion in Motion, New Hampshire Department of Health and Human Services, *https://www.dhhs.nh.gov/dphs/nhp/documents/sugar.pdf.*

> the same high. Hence, sugar is like a drug, and that's why so many of us feel caught in its grasp.[21]

Is it any wonder that I'm a sugarholic? I can't have just a little bit of sugar. I can't stop with just a small taste here and a tiny bite there. My brain goes all weird on me (sugar hijacking!), and the intense cravings start. It is so hard to say no! With great effort and commitment to my WHY over the last eighteen months, I have been able to reign in the sugar consumption. But it is still so difficult to walk by a sugar temptation and just say no. The food industry hires food scientists to study this behavior, and they create foods (and even food environments) that our brains crave at a cocaine-addiction level!

One of my favorite books from 2020 is *Limitless* by Jim Kwik. Talking about what sugar does to the brain, Jim quotes Dr. Eva Selhub:

> [She]...often likens the brain to a high-performance vehicle. Like an expensive car, she writes, your brain functions best when it gets on premium fuel. Eating high-quality foods that contain lots of vitamins, minerals, and antioxidants nourishes the brain and protects it from oxidative stress—the "waste" (free radicals) produced when the body uses oxygen, which can damage cells. She goes on to note that when your brain is forced to run on inferior fuel, it can't possibly do everything it is built to do.

This next part of her quote really hits home for me:

---

21 David Meine, *Think: Use Your Mind to Shrink Your Waistline*, (CreateSpace Independent Publishing Platform; 2nd edition April 2014), p. 80.

> Refined sugar, for example, contributes to impaired brain function, leads to inflammation, and can even cause depression (something you might want to consider the next time you reach for a tub of ice cream to contend with a tough day).[22]

Wow, the memory of that daily ice cream indulgence really stung when I read those words. Can you believe that I have spent most of my life impairing my brain function? And now I have built visceral fat around my vital organs, which is proven to lead to much higher chances of Alzheimer's or a heart attack. Sugar is truly trying to lead me to an early death or to life in a memory care facility.

It's really hard not to get frustrated—or downright angry—about the food and beverage industry. It feels like an unfair battle! I just don't understand why our government agencies and the food industry don't take a serious look at the insatiable amount of sugar each and every American is consuming. Canada and Europe banned high-fructose corn syrup years ago. Here in America, it's everywhere! It's also so difficult to eat out and find nutritious meals without lots of added sugar. Once you start really looking, you discover that almost everything is loaded with sugar, from salad dressing to meat marinades. We go about our lives blissfully ignorant and oblivious to what we're really putting in our bodies, and then we wonder why we are a nation of obese and unhealthy people.

It's pretty staggering, actually. According to the Environmental Health News, we are currently among the unhealthiest nations in the world. An astonishing 42.4% of Americans aged twenty

22 Jim Kwik, *Limitless*, (Hay House Inc.; Illustrated edition April 2020), p. 130.

and over (roughly 130 million people) are obese. The US is the sad leader of developed countries as far as how many of us have type 2 diabetes, with 11% of the population, or 34 million people. We have the third-highest mortality rate for diseases of the circulatory system in the world, including high blood pressure, and the second-highest mortality rate for heart attacks. Heart disease remains the leading cause of death in the US.[23] The disturbing list of unhealthy stats goes on and on.

I am writing this book during the COVID-19 pandemic. With all the talk and debate happening around us, there has not been much emphasis on strengthening our immune systems to fight the virus. Even with a vaccine, the very best thing we can do is to take care of our bodies. Carla and I have been vigilant about this, taking soluble vitamins C, D, and B12. We've also been so careful about what we do and don't put into our bodies. And decreasing sugar has been at the top of our list.

That's not easy when, everywhere we turn, it's sugar, sugar, and more sugar! Once you train the brain to eat a certain food or sugary snack, it is very difficult to stop. Would you ever feed a newborn baby a big apple fritter with sugar icing dripping off of it? Of course not! You'd be dealing with a sick, crying baby for hours—maybe days. We are just not designed to eat the amount of sugar in our diets today and enjoy optimum health.

Do you know what "homeostasis" means? Emeritus Professor Kelvin Rodolfo of the University of Illinois at Chicago's

---

23 Jerrold J. Heindel and Linda S. Birnbaum, "Endocrine-disrupting chemicals weaken us in our COVID-19 battle: Linda S. Birnbaum, Jerrold J. Heindel," Environmental Health News, 23 April 2020, *https://www.ehn.org/chemical-exposure-coronavirus-2645785581/an-unhealthy-nation*.

Department of Earth and Environmental Sciences provides this answer:

> Homeostasis, from the Greek words for "same" and "steady," refers to any process that living things use to actively maintain fairly stable conditions necessary for survival…[It is] how the human body maintains steady levels of temperature and other vital conditions such as the water, salt, sugar, protein, fat, calcium, and oxygen contents of the blood.[24]

Homeostasis means that our body fights to keep what it's gotten used to as its status quo, and this becomes a real challenge when it comes to sugar and the brain. As I have studied how to break a bad habit and form a new one, I came face to face with homeostasis. In simple terms, most of our habits are run at the subconscious level. Essential things like breathing, swallowing, and so many more bodily functions happen without us consciously thinking about them. Our subconscious thoughts impact our lives in much the same way, without any conscious effort. Over time, we train our brain to have nonsensical beliefs, fears, likes, and dislikes about many non-essential things.

When it comes to sugar, we have to work to retrain our brains. We have to disturb the "status quo" of old sugar habits and replace them with new, healthy habits. It takes effort, but this much I know for sure: the struggle is getting easier. It's becoming easier to keep our pantry empty of processed, sugary foods. My daily routine of foraging through the kitchen

---

24 "What is Homeostasis?" Scientific American, 3 January 2020, *https://www.scientificamerican.com/article/what-is-homeostasis/.*

and pantry to find sugary snacks has decreased dramatically. I'm getting better at saying no to foods I know cause damage and saying yes to premium fuel for my body. That's because, each day, my WHY is getting stronger. It's consciously being ingrained into my subconscious mind.

Over the last two years, I have improved my health dramatically. The sugar that was slowly killing me has been put in jail. It's not in our home. We do not search for it when we eat out. At social functions that include dinner, appetizers, and desserts, we choose "eating to live." Carla constantly researches and creates recipes that meet our optimal health goals. "Eating to live" has required me to change my taste buds. Is it hard? Sure. Is it worth it? Wholeheartedly, yes.

What does "eating to live" mean? It means that you become a scientist who is willing to find the facts about your unique body. It means you record how certain foods either remove inflammation or create pain from the esophagus down to your bowels. It means you learn the difference between visceral and subcutaneous fat and then how to decrease the bad fats along with your chances of heart disease. It means becoming your own best advocate and working hard to achieve health and wellness, and increased energy every day.

"Eating to live" means living your best life for as long as you possibly can.

I always tease individuals when they talk negatively about their doctors and health providers. I say, "Remember, these medical professionals are practicing medicine." Then I laugh and add this reminder, "Science continues to evolve, and new breakthroughs that were thought to be impossible several years ago are now modern-day miracles." I am so grateful for the researchers who continue to push the envelope to eradicate diseases and health challenges. Learning and applying all of this knowledge has resulted in a modern-day miracle in my life.

We know there are no guarantees. We don't know exactly how long we've been able to extend my life. We don't know if the cancer will return. But this much I do know: We have dramatically improved my quality of life. So far, I have remained cancer-free. We have taken my pain level from a constant eight down to less than two on a scale of one to ten. My arthritis has gone away, and my peripheral neuropathy has diminished greatly. I'm an active, involved, mentally alert, fun grandpa who plans to stay that way for many, many years to come.

Part Two of this book explains the four levels of the *Eating to Live* program and is filled with important, life-changing tips that can make a dramatic difference in your health. It is our hope that my story has resonated with you and that you have related to my crazy health journey somewhere along the line. By sharing it with you, we hope you'll be motivated to read the second half of this book. Maybe this will motivate you to wean off your medications. Maybe you will take certain foods out of your diet that are causing a leaky gut. Perhaps you will truly understand how you are creating inflammation in your body that is aggravating your arthritis, stomach issues, poor digestion, or inconsistent bowel movements. The list goes on and on. The potential for radical improvement by implementing small changes is truly great! I encourage you to join us in this journey to create your optimal health—to live your best life as long as you can—by eating to live.

Additional Information on Health in the US Today

- The US is currently one of the unhealthiest nations in the world. An astonishing 42.4% of Americans aged twenty and over (roughly 130 million people) are obese.
- The US leads developed nations in numbers of type 2 diabetes—11% of the population aged twenty to seventy-nine years; about thirty-four million people have diabetes.
- The US has the third-highest mortality rate for diseases of the circulatory system, including high blood pressure; overall, the second-highest mortality rate for heart attacks and heart disease is the leading cause of death in the US. While there has been a global decline in mortality due to circulatory disorders, the US decline is smaller than any other country measured.[25]
- The United States is among the wealthiest nations in the world, but it is far from the healthiest. Although life expectancy and survival rates in the United States have improved dramatically over the past century,

25 Jerrold J. Heindel and Linda S. Birnbaum, "Endocrine-disrupting chemicals weaken us in our COVID-19 battle," Environmental Health News, 23 April 2020, *https://www.ehn.org/chemical-exposure-coronavirus-2645785581.html?rebelltitem=1#rebelltitem1.*

Americans live shorter lives and experience more injuries and illnesses than people in other high-income countries.[26]

- When I was born, 5% of people in America were obese. Now it's 42%. That's staggering. Type 2 diabetes was very rare, but now, one out of every two Americans has prediabetes or type 2 diabetes. Six out of ten people have a chronic disease in America, and four out of ten have more than one.
- 70% of Americans are either overweight or obese (40% are obese).
- Nearly one in three Americans is suffering from diabetes or prediabetes.
- One in every four deaths in this country is caused by heart disease.[27]

Dr. Gundry observed in his book, *The Plant Paradox*:

> Starting in the mid-1960s, we have seen a rampant rise in obesity, type 1 and type 2 diabetes, autoimmune diseases, asthma, allergies and sinus conditions, arthritis, cancer, heart disease, osteoporosis, Parkinson's disease, and dementia. Not coincidentally, in the same period, there have been many seemingly imperceptible changes in our diet and in the personal care products we use. I've discovered a significant part of the answer to the mystery of why our collective health has declined,

---

26 "U.S. Health in International Perspective: Shorter Lives, Poorer Health," National Center for Biotechnology Information (NCBI), *https://www.ncbi.nlm.nih.gov/books/NBK154469/.*

27 Dr. Steven Gundry, "Dr. Mark Hyman Transcript," Dr. Gundry, 6 Mar 2020, *https://drgundry.com/dr-mark-hyman-transcript/.*

and our collective weight has risen so drastically in just a few decades—and it starts with plant proteins called lectins.[28]

28 Dr. Steven Gundry, *The Plant Paradox*, (Harper Wave; 1st edition April 2017), p. xi.

LEVEL UP: PART 2 OF EATING TO LIVE

INTRODUCTION:

THE FOUR LEVELS OF EATING TO LIVE

In Part 2 of *Eating to Live*, we will explain how you can apply the principles of functional nutrition and healthy living to your life. We take a phased approach, and you will "level up" as you progress. It's also a back-to-basics process, where you will eliminate foods from your diet, monitor and track results, and slowly add foods back in as you work your way through each level.

There are four sections in Part 2, and each section has chapters that contain the food charts for that level and additional important information about accessing optimal health. As you read, you will learn how to become your own scientist and perform your life's most important experiment: how to be the healthiest, best you!

We have created a Member Portal with additional resources for you on our website. There are many delicious and healthy recipes for each level of *Eating to Live*, videos, PDF documents, and access to virtual meetings, both live and pre-recorded.

There is also an interactive online forum, where you will have a community to connect with and a place to discuss questions or concerns and get valuable help on your health journey. As a purchaser of our book, we would like to provide you with a $10 coupon code that can be used at any time. Simply go to www.eatingtolive.com and enter code ETLMember10 to receive your discount.

In Part 1, you've read David's story with occasional insights from me, Carla. In Part Two, you will hear my voice much more frequently as I share what I've learned as a Certified Functional Nutrition Counselor. Here is a formal introduction to what I do and what functional nutrition truly is.

Meet Carla Meine, CFNC

Inspired by my many years of researching health and wellness to support and help David through his numerous health challenges, I completed a comprehensive, full-body-systems immersion program and became a Certified Functional Nutrition Counselor (CFNC). Functional nutrition uses clinical and practical tools to leverage the powers of nutrition and use "food as medicine," uncovering the root causes of problems that other practitioners may have missed. Even people who have been everywhere and tried everything are able to connect the dots and solve chronic conditions as they heal the body through individualized diet and lifestyle plans that really work.

I help clients determine which foods and lifestyle choices work best for them, and why those choices are specific to their particular physiology. As specific changes are made to diet and environment, they get to the heart of "what's going on in there" rather than masking symptoms through quick-fix solutions. I work closely with clients to help them reclaim ownership of their health and become their own health expert.

What Is Functional Nutrition?

Functional nutrition is not new or fancy, but it is the answer to many of the problems in health and healthcare today. It's a modality that works not just to support, but to educate you, the patient, about what's going on in your body, and how making uniquely targeted diet and lifestyle modifications will help you to meet your goals. Functional nutrition fills a gap between traditional medicine and the patient's needs.

A functional nutrition counselor's mission is to prevent disease occurrence and work as healers to reverse disease, anticipating problems before they happen and fine-tuning processes to offer high-quality, highly-individualized care.

LEVEL UP:
PART 2 OF *EATING TO LIVE*

Level 1

Chapter 1. Introduction to Level 1

Chapter 2. Finding Your WHY to Achieving Your Optimal Health

Chapter 3. The Eating to Live Journal

Chapter 4. The Eating to Live Meal Plan

Chapter 5. Drink More Water

Level 2

Chapter 1. An Introduction to Level 2/Level 2 Meal Plan

Chapter 2. Get Plenty of Sleep

Chapter 3. Remove NSAIDs from Your Diet

Level 3

Chapter 1. An Introduction to Level 3/Level 3 Meal Plan

Chapter 2. Train your Brain for Optimal Health

Chapter 3. Supplement Your Food with Proper Nutrition

Level 4

Chapter 1. An Introduction to Level 4/Level 4 Meal Plan

Chapter 2. Reduce Stress

Chapter 3. Exercise for a Healthy Body

Conclusion

Epilogue

Appendix I

MY WHY

Rushford Lee

I know how I'm going to die.

I know that probably sounds dramatic, but unless I get hit by a bus or have a nasty crash on my bike, cancer will eventually kill me. The writing is on the wall. It's in the cards. Let me explain.

I'm the youngest of eight siblings in a bit of a "yours, mine, and ours" situation. When my dad was fifty, and my mom was forty-six, she went to the doctor to discuss the "change of life," which she assumed was happening to her. The doctor winked and said, "You're going to have a change of life all right—you're pregnant!" When I was born, I already had eight nieces and nephews. My parents were grandparents eight times over.

As the youngest-by-far in my family, I've watched the cancer battles up close. I've already lost four of my siblings to cancer. My father lost his battle with cancer. And, at the time of this writing, two other siblings are currently dying of cancer. One might have two years to live. The other has been given six months.

I've watched them all die, and it's really ugly. One sister decided not to even fight it. She'd seen what chemotherapy did and chose not to live like that. She went into the hospital and died two weeks later, leaving her kids and young grandchildren. I've been in the room when my brothers and sisters died. I held my brother's hand as he passed. I've watched each of them suffer and struggle and ultimately lose to cancer, a vicious foe who has repeatedly wreaked havoc in our family.

The longest any of my siblings have lived is to age sixty-five. I'm now sixty years old. I've already had three malignant melanomas. So the clock is ticking, and I really do know how I'm going to die.

With my mortality staring me in the face, I decided I wanted to do anything I could to control this reality. About eighteen months ago, I started researching how not to die from cancer. I read books authored by doctors who believe that much of what causes cancer—as well as diabetes, heart problems, and a host of other ailments—are the foods we eat.

I also learned a lot through my work in branding and marketing. We do a lot of packaging design for companies, and they put a lot of things into those foods to help them stay on the shelf longer; otherwise, they lose money. Most items in a grocery store are filled with chemicals and preservatives and processed with extra sugars to taste better. All of these additives are so damaging to our health.

I've worked with meat-processing plants and poultry farms. Even the very best of them use processing techniques that destroy our bodies (and would turn your stomach if you saw them). And, although how and what these animals are fed might make sense economically, it sure doesn't make sense for our health—or theirs. They even grind up the chicken bones and feed them back to the chickens. That's not good for them, but it keeps prices down. Armed with this knowledge, I decided I had to change what I ate. I ate healthier, lost fifteen pounds, and felt a lot better.

But time passed, and it was hard to stay committed. Those fifteen pounds snuck back on as I fell back into old habits. It was around this time that I started working with David and Carla Meine on the branding for their company, Eating to Live. What they were doing resonated with me and made sense based on the reading and research I had done on my own a year before.

Hearing David's story reminded me of my own WHY for living healthy. I knew what I needed to do, but I had struggled to maintain doing it. Throughout our conversations, David would urge me to find a stronger WHY. I thought I already had a pretty good WHY and told him so. But my actions and habits told the truth.

Then, another brother died. Something in me snapped. I refused to end up like this and let cancer win! I had to do more, and I fully committed myself. I eliminated the foods I knew weren't good for me. I watched my bowels, tracked my acid levels, and made changes to my diet based on what I observed.

I don't count calories. I simply stay away from all red meat, pork, and chicken. I don't eat any cheese. I avoid all sweets and sugary beverages, and I don't eat anything that comes in a package—no processed foods. And, it's working.

With this new eating lifestyle, I lost thirty pounds and gained a new lease on life. Biking has replaced any "high" I used to get from food, and I ride about twenty miles a day, outdoors in the spring and summer and inside in a spin class through the winter. I'm in better shape now than I was last year or the year before when I'd first attempted to get healthier. I know this is because I'm no longer tasking my body with all the things that used to continually beat it up and break it down.

My new eating regimen got easier pretty quickly. Once you adapt, it's not hard at all. I'm eating all the time. I just eat good foods. Good food fills you up! My wife has been so supportive; she makes vegetarian salad dressings and cheese and a mean bean hamburger. We constantly try new things. The hardest part was changing traditions. As a business owner, I go to lunch a lot. At first, the smell of steak and fries was really hard, but now, six months later, it doesn't bother me. When my son-in-law cooks his beloved smoked beef, I might have a little, but I inevitably go home and end up sick. My body is simply not used to processing it.

You might argue that eating this way is more expensive when you're not buying the cheap processed food. My response? One heart attack could cost you $20,000 in hospital bills. Or it might cost you your life. What's the price tag on that?

It really is all about finding your WHY. You have to start with a WHY and it has to be compelling enough that you're willing to make the changes you need to make. What is finally enough to make you step back, take a look at your life, and change? What do you want to live for? What is your WHY?

My WHY is cancer. Cancer might still be the thing that kills me. But I'm doing all I can to keep it at bay. I know there are no guarantees that I've lengthened my life, but I've exponentially increased my quality of life in the meantime. By the way, I was clean at my last checkup. The doctor who has been cutting and burning growths off me for the past fifteen years, including those three malignant melanomas, said, "It's interesting how you don't seem to be having trouble anymore... Maybe we are getting a handle on things!" I nodded and smiled. Maybe we are.

LEVEL 1

CHAPTER 1

AN INTRODUCTION TO LEVEL 1

Carla Meine

In this first level of the *Eating to Live* program, you'll take the first important steps toward determining what your body needs in order to start healing and begin accessing health and wellness. We know that, chances are, you've tried other programs or solutions, but you are still living with pain, discomfort, fatigue, brain fog... The list of potential ailments is long! And, although this is not a weight-loss program, we also realize you might have some extra pounds you'd be healthier (and happier) without. A side benefit of *Eating to Live* is that those pounds come off as you focus on healing your gut.

Level 1 is, as my amazing teacher Andrea Nakayama likes to say, all about "clearing the muddy waters." You get to become the scientist, and your body is the lab experiment—the most important experiment you'll ever conduct, with potentially life-saving results. You'll get to discover for yourself what foods work for you and which don't. This process of discovery takes time; exactly how much time depends on the individual. You will need to commit to at least thirty days to see if you start feeling better. Those with more chronic issues will take longer. You'll gather the evidence, and then you get to decide what is working for you.

As a functional nutrition coach, the most common question I get is, "What should I eat if I want to be healthy?" This is a tricky question and not nearly as clear-cut as you might think. That's because the answer is highly individualized, and what you should eat might be completely different from what someone else should eat. The job of a functional nutritionist is to help you find the nutrition lifestyle that is perfect for you.

It's also important to define what "healthy" means. So many people view this through the exclusive lens of weight. They think being healthy means maintaining a certain number on the scale. This is partially true. It is possible, however, to be thin and still be remarkably unhealthy. Some doctors tell stories of skinny wives who bring their overweight husbands in for treatment when the wives are just as sick as their husbands, and are taking just as many medications. But because they're thin, they think they're healthy.

The other day, I was talking with my kids and, during the course of the conversation, I said, "I am the healthiest I've ever been in my life that I can remember." And I meant it! Maybe when I was a lot younger, I was healthier than I am now, but of the last twenty-five years, I truly feel better than I've ever felt. My kids, however, were shocked.

They said, "You think you're healthier now than when you were doing triathlons, mom? Because, man, you were super fit then!"

And I said, without hesitation, "Yes! I absolutely think I'm healthier now—even with an additional twenty pounds—than I was then. I might've been faster and leaner and able to lift heavier weights, but I wasn't healthier."

And it's true! I was super fit during those competitive years. I looked amazing, at 5'9" and 125 pounds, wearing the little triathlon outfits and working out all the time. But I wasn't healthy. My digestive system wasn't working as well as it is now, and I didn't feel as good as I do now. So, here at *Eating to Live*, we define "optimal health" as achieving the best possible health for your body's individual genetic composition.

Digestion Matters

I could write the rest of this book about the digestive system and the importance of a healthy gut. Don't worry, I won't! But I could, because it truly is that important. But for our purposes, I want to give you just a basic understanding of why this matters so much. Knowing makes a big difference, because if you don't clearly understand why it is so important to make these changes, you probably won't be willing to stick to them.

Here's the truth: Every bit of your health—all of it—stems back to or is rooted in digestive issues. This is not an exaggeration. The health of your gut is implicated in every single system in your entire body.

You're probably reading this and thinking that has to be a false, overstated claim, but it's absolutely true. Stay with me here. I'm going to explain it as succinctly as I can, but it's important you understand how your body works. Comprehending this will really help you stay motivated and committed to fueling your body better.

Most of my education about food is around what food does to your digestive system and your immune system. These are two areas that we have seen fail in David, and his leaky gut has subsequently led to many, if not all, of his health issues. When the digestive and immune systems are getting the nutrition they need, they are amazing at identifying foreign objects and eliminating them before they can do any damage. When they are fed foods that break down the small intestine wall and let food particles in that shouldn't be there—foods that contain sugar and gluten, for example—we see the body go on full attack mode. When this occurs for extended periods of time, the result can be diabetes, heart disease, autoimmune diseases, and even cancer.

Our bodies come with this amazing immune system. It is a sophisticated and dynamic network that is constantly working to identify foreign invaders (figuring out what is self vs. non-self, or nowadays, with all the additional toxins and non-natural substances we deal with, self vs. dangerous other). Once the danger is identified, the immune system initiates a series of communications and activates the proper attack, all in an attempt to keep each one of your body systems healthy and functional.

Did you know that the number-one immune system defense is your skin? But that isn't limited to the skin on the outside of your body. It is also the skin on the inside of your body, or the "wet tissue." This includes the area around your eyes, your respiratory system, your reproductive system, and, most importantly, your digestive system.

There's a pretty good explanation back in Chapter 10 of Section 1 about the basics of our digestive system, including its important functions and the damage we so often unknowingly incur through diet and environment. I encourage you to take a look at that information again. It's vital to understand that the gut truly is the gateway to good health.

It's also important to understand that your gut is your body's "second brain." That's right—although it can't do math problems or write poetry, you really do have a "brain" in your gut. According to an article on the brain-gut connection by Johns Hopkins Medicine:

> If you've ever "gone with your gut" to make a decision or felt "butterflies in your stomach" when nervous, you're likely getting signals from an unexpected source: your second brain. Hidden in the walls of the digestive system, this "brain in your gut" is revolutionizing medicine's understanding of the links between digestion, mood, health, and even the way you think. Scientists call this little brain the enteric nervous system (ENS). And it's not so little. The ENS is two thin layers of more than 100 million nerve cells lining your gastrointestinal tract from the esophagus to rectum.[29]

Your gut and your brain are in constant communication. And the pressure is on your gut: "In a single day, the gastrointestinal tract (your digestive system) has to make more decisions than

29 "The Brain-Gut Connection," John Hopkins Medicine, *https://www.hopkinsmedicine.org/health/wellness-and-prevention/the-brain-gut-connection.*

the rest of the body's immune system makes in its lifetime."[30] The science and medical world are being revolutionized as their understanding of this brain-gut connection grows, and they're beginning to realize it affects our brains, our moods, our behavior, and our health.

"In the last decade, we've discovered that the gut has an outsize effect on the way our brain functions," explains Jim Kwik, author of *Limitless*. "One can liken it to the way a tree functions. The roots in the ground are drawing up vital nutrients and water from the soil as well as communicating with the other plants. Those nutrients are then brought up into the body of the tree, fortifying and building the trunk, and giving the tree what it needs to sprout new leaves each spring, which in turn gather light, another energy source."[31]

There are several things we do and consume that impact the brain-gut access and, therefore, adversely affect our immune system's ability to perform as we need it to. These things include:

- Pollutants and toxins
- Alcohol consumption
- Smoking
- Fried foods
- Sugar
- Lack of nutrients
- Chronic infection
- Drugs (painkillers and antibiotics)

---

30 Professor Lloyd Meir, quoted by Andrea Nakayama in the Immune System Intensive, May-June 2020.

31 Jim Kwik, *Limitless*, (Hay House Inc.; Illustrated edition April 2020), p. 39.

- Lack of sleep
- Chronic stress

We will be addressing many items on this list as we work toward achieving optimal health. But one of the most important things we can do to positively affect our health is to clean up our diet and optimize our digestion. There is no way to bypass this step. The old adage of "junk in equals junk out" is true! Everything we put in our mouths has a direct effect, for good or for bad, on our body—especially our own self-defense system.

Andrea Nakayama, founder of the Functional Nutrition Alliance, says, "Of all the body's systems, the immune system responds most sensitively to subtle changes in our nutritional status.... Impaired immunity is a portal for infectious disease states, which then raises the need for nutritional intervention. Essentially, optimal immunity requires optimal nutrition."[32] Dietary cleanup is absolutely essential for good health!

As we begin identifying what your specific body's nutritional needs are, we will start by eliminating foods from your diet, then slowly add them back in as you track how your body reacts. What your body can tolerate will be very individual to you; however, there are some foods that are very problematic for everyone. Sugar and gluten are two of the worst culprits.

We understand that giving up these foods will not be easy. We get that the thought of living without either of them may feel overwhelming. But before you throw in the towel and quit before you've even started, I'd like to take a few pages and give you a mini-course on what sugar and gluten do to your

32 Andrea Nakayama, Immune System Intensive, May-June 2020.

system. Once you understand what they're doing each time you consume them, then you'll understand why you need to avoid them as much as possible.

Villain #1: Sugar

In a previous chapter, David talked about his sugar addiction. I loved how real and honest he was about the problem he has dealt with. When we got married, I couldn't believe the amount of sugar he would consume on a daily basis. It shocked me that someone who seemed so healthy and appeared to be so fit would do that to his body. The sad thing was that, instead of influencing him to eat less sugar, I joined him and started eating more sugar. He would have all the treats around our house, and before I knew it, I was eating them right alongside him. I figured since I was joining him in training for triathlons, that meant I could eat all the junk food, and I'd be fine. From a weight standpoint, that was true, but as I said before, when you're trying to achieve your optimal health, it's a real menace.

So let's talk about what sugar does to the digestive system, how it affects our immune system, and why we can get really sick. In some cases, the damage can be so bad that we will have to live with it the rest of our lives, and ultimately, we end up dying from it.

When it comes to the list of "immune system villains," sugar is at the very top of the list. Sugar directly affects your immune function by suppressing the production of white blood cells. White blood cells are key to our health, as they defend us against various pathogens, like viruses, bacteria, and parasites. There are five different types of white blood cells, each with its own specific protective assignment, but for our purposes, we'll keep it simple and describe them all as little trash collectors that are trained to be on the lookout for dangerous molecules. These cells are like little PacMans in your blood. As soon as they detect any foreign components in your body, they gobble them up.

A healthy body produces 2,000 immune cells every minute. You have approximately 2 million of these PacMan white blood cells circulating in your bloodstream at any given time. They stay busy and work really hard around the clock. But, these cells actually shrink when they're exposed to sugar! And, sugar keeps white blood cells from fulfilling their assigned responsibilities and protecting our immune system.

According to Nakayama, "Three ounces of sugar[33] in any form results in about a 50% reduction in white blood cell activity for anywhere from one to five hours."[34] ("Sugar in any form" here is referring to any form of processed sugar.) It's also important to realize that cancer cells feed off sugar. All cells in our bodies do, but the fast-growing cells like cancer will take all of the sugar they can and use it to proliferate.

Refined sugar is actually an anti-nutrient. Let me explain: When we consume processed sugar, which contains no fiber, minerals, proteins, fats, or enzymes, not only are we eating empty calories, but our body has to borrow vital nutrients from healthy cells in order to metabolize it. Calcium, sodium, potassium, magnesium, thiamine, chromium, zinc, B vitamins, and other minerals all get "robbed" from our healthy cells so that the body can biochemically break down and absorb the

---

33 That's just under 7 tablespoons of granulated sugar.

34 Andrea Nakayama, Immune System Intensive, May-June 2020.

sugar. So that sugar is depleting our bodies of vital nutrients, which is particularly worrisome, as our overall mineral levels are typically already pretty depleted. Also, like gluten, sugar causes inflammation in the body, and inflammation causes pain and chronic, long-term health issues.

This is where nutrition really matters; the better our nutrition, the healthier our immune cells (and our ability to produce them) will be. When we're exposed to things that compromise our immune system, like sugar, we are seriously compromising our health.

Villain #2: Gluten

The next food villain that causes a variety of health issues is gluten. Once again, David got real with you about his addiction to gluten and how hard it has been to get rid of it in his diet. It's understandable. It is hard to imagine a life without bread, not to mention the many other foods that contain gluten as well.

Here's the problem with gluten: Gluten really affects the gut-brain connection, because gluten and casein don't simply move through your bloodstream. These peptides are small enough that they are able to cross the blood-brain barrier.

Remember those lectins, the dagger-like proteins that are so good at getting through the gut wall, which we discussed in Chapter 10 of Part 1? Once they get through that wall, they wreak all sorts of havoc. Your immune system goes on the attack no differently than if those peptides were harmful viruses or bacteria. As if that weren't bad enough, those peptides are also highly addictive. In fact, they fit in the same category as opiates.

As you read this definition of opiates, see if it sounds similar to how you feel when you eat a fresh, warm roll or a thick slice of homemade bread:

> An opiate is a narcotic that blocks the transmission of pain messages to the brain. Opioids also tend to induce euphoria by affecting the brain regions that mediate pleasure—leaving feelings of warmth, drowsiness, and contentment. Opioids relieve stress and discomfort by resting a relaxed detachment from pain, desires, and activity.[35]

Sound familiar? And there's more. Dr. William Davis, a renowned cardiologist and author, tells us that modern wheat is an opiate:

> I don't mean that wheat is an opiate in the sense that you like it so much that you feel you are addicted. Wheat is truly addictive. Wheat is addictive in the sense that it comes to dominate thoughts and behaviors. Wheat is addictive in the sense that, if you don't have any for several hours, you start to get nervous, foggy, tremulous, and start desperately seeking out another "hit" of crackers, bagels, or bread, even if it's the few stale three-month-old crackers at the bottom of the box. Wheat is addictive in the sense that there is a distinct withdrawal syndrome characterized by overwhelming fatigue, mental "fog," inability to exercise, even depression that lasts several days, occasionally several weeks. Wheat is addictive in the sense that the withdrawal process can

---

35 Andrea Nakayama, Immune System Intensive, May-June 2020.

> be provoked by administering an opiate-blocking drug such as naloxone or naltrexone.

Davis goes on to explain that the high we get from wheat isn't the same as the high of heroin, morphine, or OxyContin. "This opiate, while it binds to the opiate receptors of the brain, doesn't make us high; it makes us hungry."[36]

That hunger helps explain another issue—weight gain. Dr. Gundry explains:

> Wheat is addictive, acting like an opiate in your brain. Like most people, you tolerate its ill effects because you are addicted to it. In addition to its addictive properties, wheat presents another huge problem for us—it actively promotes weight gain. According to the Centers for Disease Control, 70.7% of American adults are overweight, and of those, almost 38% are obese. Twenty years ago, less than 20% were obese. Sadly, being overweight is the new normal, and lectins (wheat gluten) play a large role in this obesity crisis.[37]

As we've already discussed, chronic inflammation is the cause of so many of our problems, including heart disease, diabetes, cancer, arthritis, and bowel diseases like Crohn's disease and ulcerative colitis. It can also lead to autoimmune disorders, such as rheumatoid arthritis and lupus.

---

36 Dr. William Davis, "Wheat is an opiate," Wheat Belly Blog, 17 April 2012, *https://www.wheatbellyblog.com/2012/04/wheat-is-an-opiate/.*

37 Dr. Steven Gundry, MD, *The Plant Paradox*, (Harper Wave; 1st edition, 2017), p. 42.

Research confirms that gluten reeks with guilt when it comes to inflammation, and it's part of a vicious cycle:

> Without question, today, there has been an explosion of three major inflammation factors: gluten sensitivity, leaky gut (or intestinal permeability), and autoimmunity. Additionally, it appears that these three factors combine to create vicious cycles, leading to various ailments and symptoms. For example, gluten sensitivity leads to leaky gut, or leaky gut development leads to gluten sensitivity, and both gluten sensitivity and leaky gut have been shown to be major triggers for various autoimmune responses. Also, the inflammatory response of autoimmunity promotes tight gap junction breakdown and intestinal permeability, and gluten sensitivity.[38]

These wheat issues are highly amplified by our wheat production processes in the US, by the way. You might not experience all of the same wheat-related issues if you eat wheat products produced elsewhere. Wheat grown and produced in America, however, is a major threat to our health.

Here is a brief synopsis of why: US grain production includes the hybridization and deamidation of the grain, specifically of the gliadin proteins or gluten. Deamidation means that the amide, a chemical group, has been removed from the original protein structure. With these modifications, the new proteins are very similar to other tissues in our body, especially that of

38 D. Kharrazian, "The Gluten, Leaky Gut, Autoimmune Connection. Apex Energetics lecture," 16 Mar 2013.

brain tissue. This is one reason why we see such a prevalence of memory issues and brain fog with autoimmune conditions.

The modified protein also induces intestinal inflammation (think celiac or leaky gut). So when we eat these modified, man-made gliadin (gluten) peptides, they're able to cross the weakened barrier system in the gut into the bloodstream. Our immune system tries to recognize it. It works on developing antibodies to defend us from this new invader. And it remembers this invader, so the next time it encounters anything that looks similar, it attacks again. Because these proteins are so similar to self-tissue, like brain tissue, we end up with a chronic, constant attack on the self. This shows up as chronic inflammation. But it's really our dedicated, overworked immune system trying to put out what it perceives as a "fire."[39]

This is exactly why David continued to have such struggles, even after cutting out almost all gluten from his diet. Remember that yummy sourdough bread? To really start to heal, to get rid of the chronic pain and inflammation he was living with, he had to give up gluten completely. If you're thinking to yourself, "But I hardly eat gluten anymore," the "hardly" counts more than you think!

According to Nakayama,

> 95% gluten-free does not mean 95% protected from gluten. It means 0% protected from gluten. Is it worse? Yes. The cumulative situation will lead more quickly to that later stage of disease. But any at all is not

39 Nore Hoogstad, "What's Wrong with Gluten," Gutsy by Nutrition, 18 February 2019, *https://gutsybynutrition.com.au/gutsy-by-nutrition-blog/2019/2/14/whats-wrong-with-gluten.*

> going to allow for the conditions of healing, and the circumstances for slowing down the progression of disease will not be present.[40]

How Level 1 Works

Level 1 is designed to remove foods that could be causing you grief. The only way to know which foods your body can and can't handle is to first take them out of your diet. Then, as you continue through Levels 2, 3, and 4 of *Eating to Live*, you will slowly add foods back as you track results. As you do this, you'll be able to see clear patterns and undisputable data, and then you will get to decide what is best for your life and your health.

We only get one body! Our bodies are amazing and do incredible things, but their ability to perform is impacted every day by the world around us. We can't control all of our environment, but there are many things we can control. Eating nutritious meals and fueling our bodies properly is an important choice we can make every day. It's a choice that's a lot easier to make if we remain focused on our purpose and we remember why we choose to do it.

David wrote the following chapter to help you determine your WHY, which will be integral to your success.

"We don't get burned out because of what we do. We get burned out because we forget why we do it."

—AUTHOR UNKNOWN

---

40 Andrea Nakayama, Immune System Intensive, May-June 2020.

CHAPTER 2

FINDING YOUR WHY TO ACHIEVING YOUR OPTIMAL HEALTH

David Meine

What is the hardest thing you have ever done or experienced in your life? Mine was going through chemotherapy for my bladder cancer. The fear I had about facing the possible horrible side effects of chemo was indescribable, but I chose to do it. I found the strength to face these fears and take on chemo because of my WHY. If my WHY hadn't been strong enough, there is no way I could have done it. Gratefully, my fears ended up being unfounded, and although chemo was terrifically difficult, I did not experience the side effects I had dreaded. Because I knew my WHY, I am now living cancer-free.

Asking yourself, "Why am I doing this?" is so important—and difficult!—for most of us. But it is key. It is of epic importance to find your WHY!

I have wanted to live to be at least 100 years old for as long as I can remember. You must be asking yourself why that would sound so appealing to me. To be honest, I love life. I absolutely love my wife and family. I definitely need to reach the age of ninety-five so that I can celebrate fifty years with my beautiful wife, Carla. I feel lucky to live in a time that is filled with fascinating scientific and technological advances happening every day. Fishing and golfing with family and friends bring me such lasting happiness. I plan to do that until I am well past 100 years old. I want to be the oldest guy out on the course and the old man on the river still reeling in big, beautiful trout!

When I talk to friends or acquaintances about my hobbies, it's interesting to see if we align at all. My favorite hobby is fishing. When I ask the question, "Do you like to fish?" (I am always looking for fishing buddies), within a heartbeat, I know if they do or don't. If they are passionate about it, they look me in the eye and start jabbering. If it's not on their radar, they will look down and pause before they speak. At that moment, I know that fishing is not one of their interests, and that's okay.

Running into a shy person revs up my curiosity. With a smile on my face, I just start asking questions until I find what they are passionate about. Inevitably, I ask them why they are so passionate about the particular hobby, sport, author, video game, or whatever I have uncovered. At this point, they no longer seem shy. I can visibly see their energy increase. Their eyes light up. They stand up straighter. They smile as they launch passionately into their WHY.

What's my point? If you have a strong WHY that has been clearly thought out, that is something you are passionate about, that excites you, your chances of success in replacing a negative behavior and creating a positive habit are very high. The struggle comes with the doubts that others have planted at the very core of our subconscious. Emotional eating is one of those negative habits that is so destructive. In our past business, I worked with so many men and women who would lose over 100 pounds, only to have a negative situation arise in their life. Then they resorted to old habits, believing the only way to cope was by eating and drinking 5,000 calories a day through the crisis. Within a few months, they put all the weight back on.

Losing over 100 pounds takes a year and a lot of hard work! What happened to those individuals' WHY statements when they faltered and put all that weight back on? What was that subconscious nuclear bomb that would blow away all that work and brain retraining? Let's get into the nitty-gritty details and figure out WHY.

In 2013, my friend Jacob challenged me to read Simon Sinek's book, *Start with Why*. He had been contracted to provide videos for the company where I was the CEO/Founder; however, he told me that he would not follow through on his contract until our executive team read this particular book.

"Because," Jacob explained, looking me intently in the eyes, "I honestly believe that, as a company, you don't know your WHY." I was a bit stunned at such strong-arm tactics, to be honest. But Jacob was right. As Sinek says, "People don't buy what you do; they buy why you do it." Really pinpointing our WHY for doing what we were doing as a company made a big difference.

Sinek has a famous TED Talk called "Start with Why" that I encourage you to watch.[41] In that presentation, he shares the following diagram:

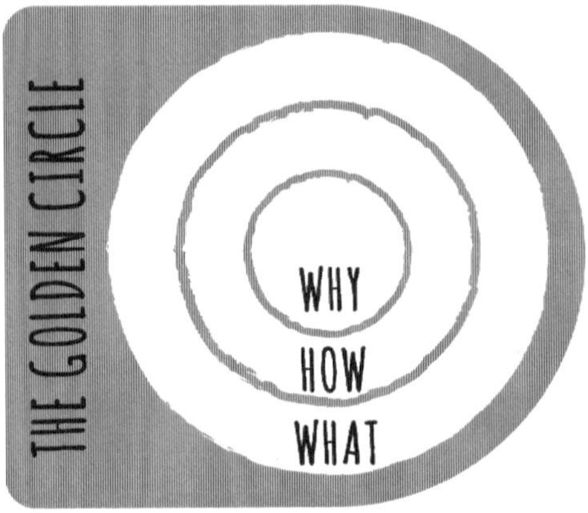

Sinek, Simon. *Start with Why*. Mar. 10, 2014.

He calls this "The Golden Circle." Simon uses this little idea to explain that everyone, no matter what the specific situation is, pretty much knows their WHAT. They know what to do. In the case of a typical New Year's resolution, the WHAT would be to lose fifteen pounds. Simon then explains that some people know how to do it. In this same example, they might adjust their diet by eliminating unhealthy carbs and sugar, or they start tracking calories or add a new workout regimen.

But very few people really know why they do what they do. If the WHY isn't clear enough and meaningful enough, then when the first sugar craving hits, or when it's late at night,

41 Simon Sinek, "Start with Why," TED, September 2009, *https://www.ted.com/talks/simon_sinek_how_great_leaders_inspire_action?language=en.*

and you're hungry enough that caring about your new goal is harder, or you have a crisis at work, and you're super stressed out, the HOW and the WHAT go out the window. If we work from the outside in, working from the WHAT to the HOW and only then to the WHY, we go from the clearest to the fuzziest thing. The most effective people and organizations all think, act, and communicate from the inside out. They start with and keep their WHY at their core.

When I first became acquainted with Sinek's ideas, I was writing a book and focusing on self-sabotage, which are behaviors or thought patterns that hold us back and prevent us from doing what we want to do. This is something we're all probably well acquainted with since we all experience it at one time or another in our lives. Let's take those New Year's resolutions as an example. Many folks feel really ambitious and want to change their life for the better at the beginning of January. I am one of them. I start out highly motivated and write down several goals I'm committed to achieving during the year. But then a few months go by, and those goals are already forgotten. Why do we do that? We start out with great intentions and then lose momentum.

Remember in the previous chapter, I talked about the brain striving for homeostasis? The brain literally is the cause of self-sabotage. Setting a goal is really hard for the brain. The brain says, "I know you want a new behavior, but guess what—you spent years training me to have your current behavior, and I am not convinced that you really want to change."

Honestly, it is so frustrating to get people to understand that they are not going crazy. They tell me, "This should not be this hard!" and they smack themselves in the head. But the truth is, it can take much longer than you think to form a new habit. The brain will not want to cooperate with your new goal of a behavior change. We used to believe it took at least four weeks to ingrain a new behavior. Now, however, research says the average time required is sixty-six days,[42] and sometimes, it might actually take much longer. You have to literally prove to the brain that you really do intend to change. This is the way our brains are designed; otherwise, you'd be changing behaviors every day, and you'd be a mess! That's the purpose of homeostasis, even though it can make positive change difficult. The brain holds onto a subconscious behavior until it knows you are serious.

This is the reason that I have had such a hard time changing ingrained, or what I call "trained" behaviors. Once we are alerted from the conscious mind that a behavior is causing negative consequences, it is the subconscious, automatic-habit neurons that baffle us. We ask ourselves, "Why is it so difficult to change when the conscious mind clearly knows that there is a problem?" Due to homeostasis, the conscious mind and the subconscious mind frequently fight against each other.

That's why The Golden Circle by Simon Sinek is such a great visual—three circles and three simple words. "What," "how," and "why" are the conversations that you must have with your brain. Working from his model as a starting place, I have developed an easy and effective way to implement this. First, it is so critical that you write down the behavior that you want to change. This should typically cause an intense emotional response. Second, you have to figure out your WHY from that

42 "How long does it take to form a habit?" University College London, 4 August 2009, *https://www.ucl.ac.uk/news/2009/aug/how-long-does-it-take-form-habit.*

emotion. After that, it should be fairly straightforward to define your HOW and WHAT statements. The more specific you can get, the better.

This is how the Why-How-What Worksheet[43] looks:

1. **BehaviortoModifyorChange:**____________________
2. **WHY:** ____
3. **HOW:** ____
4. **WHAT:** _______________________________________

Sometimes your HOW and/or your WHAT will require multiple line items. Let me give you an example of one of my own Why-How-What Worksheets.

1. **Behavior to Modify or Change:** I want to stop taking NSAIDs (Advil, Naproxen, Aleve).
2. **WHY:** I want to heal my leaky gut so that I no longer experience excruciating pain.
3. **HOW:** I will no longer take any form of NSAIDs.
4. **WHAT:** Throw away all bottles of Advil, Naproxen, and Aleve that are in the house, sports bags, vehicles, purses, etc.
   WHAT: Decrease sugar, breads, and pastries that cause inflammation, so I don't need the NSAIDs.
   WHAT: When I'm in pain, instead of reaching for ibuprofen, I will distract myself by going for a walk, doing mindful meditation and visualization exercises, watching a movie, playing a game, listening to a book, etc., in order to change my focus.

43 Find at *eatlingtolive.com/book/.*

Notice how, in this example, the WHAT required three separate entries. And it could potentially include more. The HOW and the WHAT support your WHY, and the more specific they are, the better prepared you'll be. But, if your WHY is shaky, it won't matter how good your HOW and WHAT are. Your WHY is what sustains you when times get tough.

When I was told by the first doctor that I needed to give up NSAIDs, he didn't give me any reason why. He just said, "I would recommend that you give up NSAIDs." It was almost impossible for me to maintain motivation to stay off these drugs I was so addicted to.

The second doctor explained the cause and effect of taking ibuprofen—that it was causing inflammation and creating a vicious cycle. Although getting off NSAIDs was still incredibly difficult, I now had the beginnings of a WHY. Since then, I have done additional study and been shocked to learn how harmful these medicines are, and I am now much more informed about how they are actually causing my leaky gut. This knowledge has exponentially fueled my WHY.

The brain requires a mental picture of *why* the bad habit needs to change. Essentially, you start with an emotion and then drill down from there. For me, I was emotionally discouraged and debilitated by daily pain. I knew if I could find a healthy habit that would decrease the pain, the gratitude I would feel would be empowering. I came up with three WHATs and one HOW to do this. If my WHY is not strong enough, I will not follow through on the HOW and WHAT for very long. In my case, I could continue to eat the gluten and the sugar and live with the pain. Or, I could decide that I no longer want to deal with chronic pain and determine to eliminate those foods from my diet.

But, if my WHY is not strong enough, the next time someone is eating a toasted coconut donut in front of me and offers me one, I'll cave. My taste buds *really* love a good donut! However, if I remember that the donut is not only the bad guy that causes me bodily pain, but is also the cause of the visceral fat I have around my organs that leads to heart disease and Alzheimer's, I might find the willpower to say, "No, thanks!" to that temporary donut pleasure. If we give in day after day, we will either quit or be forced to strengthen our WHY. The WHY is what makes it personal.

Let's take this a step further. Going back to the previous example, with my three WHAT statements above, which behavior do you think would be the easiest to accomplish? You might say that throwing away the NSAIDs would be the easiest unless you are in a lot of pain, which I definitely was at the time. Regardless of pain levels, decreasing sugar, breads, and pastries are pretty daunting behavior changes in and of themselves.

To be successful, we have to think about each WHAT and see if they will create barriers to success or traumatic failures that make you give up on the original WHY. Ask yourself, "Do I have too many WHAT statements, or not enough?" You have your brain fully engaged when you are working in Sinek's Golden Circle.

Accountability Is Key

Hang in there with me and let's take this one step further. The ultimate key to successfully creating positive changes is through accountability. In any goal-setting exercise, success or failure depends on your daily accountability review. Our brains have to clearly see we are constantly thinking about the WHY, HOW, and WHAT. We can't change behavior with just a wish. Being accountable to our WHY is more than a wish, and leads to true and effective change.

My favorite way to do this is through good, old-fashioned journaling, either the old-school way with pen and paper or on an electronic device. Your system should be very easy and only take a few minutes to do. Writing it down and keeping yourself accountable helps immensely. Keep it simple, but find something that works for you. The sample below shows how I journaled each day by using checklists and reporting on my phone when I was working on eliminating NSAIDs.

Date:	
Behavior change:	I want to stop taking NSAIDS, "Advil, Naproxen, Aleve"
WHY statement:	I want to stop suffering from my leaky gut
HOW statement:	Did I take NSAIDS today? YES____ NO____
WHAT statement:	Did I eat sugar today? YES____ NO____
WHAT statement:	Did I eat bread today? YES____ NO____
Incremental results:	Did I feel any decrease in pain today? YES____ NO____
What was challenging for me today:	
Write down one positive result from my efforts today:	

Checking in with yourself at the end of the day not only keeps you accountable, but it helps you to realize the good that is happening, even if it is in incremental doses. Seeing this will strengthen your WHY, which in turn strengthens your motivation. Doing this experiment day after day will begin to wake up the subconscious mind to the fact that you really want to change behavior and create a new habit. Seeing even small improvements as you remain accountable to yourself each day helps convince your brain that homeostasis needs to alter and that you really do intend to make a change.

I'd like to share another significant example of this with you. Throughout the first half of this book, I shared that, although I visited many doctors over many years, it wasn't until Dr. Gundry that anyone ever talked to me about my diet. Instead, all of those other doctors simply prescribed medications based on whatever symptoms I was currently having. The number of medications that I was taking for pain, heartburn, peripheral neuropathy, swollen prostate, ED, arthritis pain, and my list of ailments goes on, simply continued to increase. Here is another shocker: In all of those years, I have never had a doctor tell me that I needed to stop taking a prescription. Why is that?

When Dr. Gundry meets with older patients (I classify myself as one of those) at his restorative medicine practice, they are taking, on average, anywhere between seven and fifteen medications. And here I thought my five daily medications were outrageous! One of his main goals is to help his patients, through diet and natural supplements, to be able to dismiss their dependence on medications that typically have serious side effects.

I knew it was important for me to get off the other medications I was taking, in addition to the NSAIDs. One of these medications was Cymbalta, or as it is known generically, Duloxetine. I had started taking this medication for my severe neuropathy back when I was battling bladder cancer. At my yearly appointment with my neurologist, I'd told him that I'd been dealing with a lot of physical pain. During that conversation, I explained that I was getting really discouraged, and because I felt some trust in this doctor, I even confided that I was starting to wonder if the battle was worth fighting.

His response was, "David, I think we need to add a medication to work with the Lyrica that you are currently taking." Without any further explanation, he proceeded to write out a prescription for Cymbalta. I asked what this drug would specifically do. He stated that it would decrease my pain and decrease my discouragement. He did not warn me about the common side effects, which include dry mouth, headache, and nausea, or the possibility of more serious (and sometimes fatal) side effects, such as abnormal bleeding, liver damage, and suicidal thoughts and behaviors.

At the time, I had no idea that my increased levels of pain were from all the sugar I was drinking in my supposed "cancer-busting" juice diet. The medicine did seem to help with my pain and the dark thoughts I'd been having. But years passed, and this medication was never discussed again. No one from his office has ever said it was time to stop taking it. Neither he nor his staff ever encouraged me that it was time to wean off the medicine. After seeing Dr. Gundry, however, I had gotten myself off of Advil, Naproxen, Aleve, and Lortab. I'd even gotten off of my small "dailies" like Tums and Pepto Bismol. The Cymbalta (Duloxetine) was next in line.

I used the same Why-How-What Worksheet formula to modify this behavior.

1. **Behavior to Modify or Change:** I want to stop taking Cymbalta or its generic form, Duloxetine.
2. **WHY:** I want to stop my dependence on Duloxetine so I can optimize my overall health.
3. **HOW:** Stop taking Duloxetine.
4. **WHAT:** Meet with the doctor to find out how to wean off the drug without adverse side effects.
   WHAT: Monitor any pain changes.
   WHAT: Monitor and acknowledge any emotional changes each night with my journaling.

I am happy to say that I followed the process, stuck with it, and was able to stop taking a drug that has serious side effects. Since then, I have also been able to eliminate Lyrica, which worked together with the Duloxetine to diminish the burning pain of neuropathy (as well as a long laundry list of other ailments). Weaning off Lyrica was a major win, and I'm lucky I didn't have side effects that affected my mental health, as so many people do. It's so upsetting to me that no one addressed reducing the inflammation in my body before giving me this highly addictive and life-changing drug. (Pfizer makes billions a year off the millions of scripts written for Lyrica.)

I am now down to just Finasteride, which is a medication I take for my enlarged prostate that has plagued me for over twenty years. I was hesitant about including these sensitive issues, but my goal is to help others through sharing my story, and millions of men are affected by prostate and ED issues.[44] Since beginning my *Eating to Live* diet protocol, I no longer have ED. It's been a dramatic change and solved a problem I'd been dealing with since my early fifties. And Dr. Gundry assures me that the supplementation regimen I'm now on will solve the prostate issues, so when I have my yearly bladder cancer exam, we will see if it is possible to stop taking Finasteride. Perhaps by the time I write the epilogue of this book, I will have an update and be able to say I am now off all my prescription medication and living without pain. I'm almost there!

It has taken over two years to make such a dramatic change to my health and get myself off all of these drugs. It has been difficult to get my brain on board. The ever-present battle between the conscious mind and the subconscious mind is so fascinating. The challenge is exacerbated when we are putting chemicals, foods, beverages, and medications that affect our focus into our bodies.

Where Is Our Focus?

Let's talk about how focusing on WHY is really about learning how to focus the brain. Consider this quote by Paulo Coelho:

> Whenever you want to achieve something, keep your eyes open, concentrate, and make sure you know

44 Five percent of men 40 and older have complete erectile dysfunction. Mild and moderate ED affects about 10% of men per decade of life, (so 50% of men in their 50s, etc.). Many older men also have other health conditions that require medication that causes ED. Source: *https://www.uwhealth.org/urology/erectile-dysfunction-ed/20537.*

> exactly what it is you want. No one can hit their target with their eyes closed.[45]

Following the Golden Circle of WHY, HOW, and WHAT creates the ability to focus on changing negative behaviors into positive superpowers. One of the best books I read last year was *Limitless* by Jim Kwik, which discusses unlocking our potential and building an exceptional life through brain training. Kwik states:

> One of my core beliefs is that human potential is one of the only infinite resources we have in the world. Most everything else is finite, but the human mind is the ultimate superpower—there is no limit to our creativity, imagination, determination, or ability to think, reason, or learn.[46]

Let's talk about a superpower we all can achieve: a highly focused brain.

A Story about Focus

There's a beautiful bridge that is part of a trail I frequently ride. I currently ride three to four days a week to work on losing the 5.29 pounds of visceral fat that are still plaguing me. Luckily, I love to ride, and it's not only good exercise—it's good therapy!

In this picture, you'll notice there are three possible entrances onto this bridge. Although my average riding speed during my rides is 15.4 mph, at this particular point, I am descending

---

45 Paulo Coelho, *The Devil and Miss Prym*, (HarperOne, 2006).

46 Jim Kwik, *Limitless*, (Hay House Inc.; Illustrated edition April 2020), p. xxiii.

from a hill and usually clock around 22 mph. In a car, that doesn't seem very fast, but on a bike where your whole body is exposed, and one little clip can take you out, that is speedy! My question for you is, which of the three entry points would you take at 22 mph?

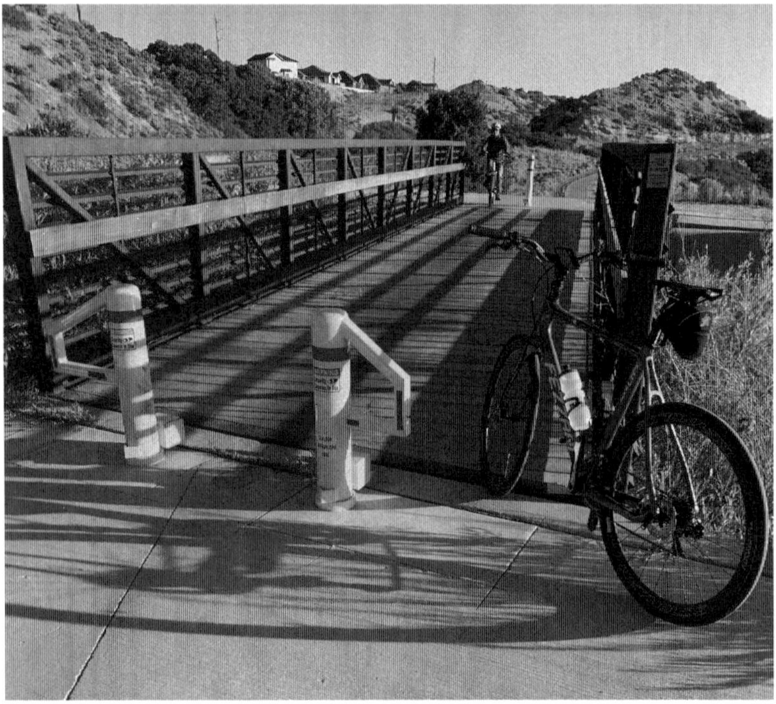

I believe that most of you would eliminate the far left, especially if another rider is approaching. That leaves the middle and the right side. You will notice that on the right and left entry points, there are bars protruding from the posts. It's deceiving, but all three entry points are actually equal distance apart.

90% of the time, I go through the middle entry. Even though it looks bigger, it's still very intimidating. Riding between obstacles at high speeds made me very nervous, and I used to slow down before entering, seeing as how I value all of my skin and I prefer my bones intact. All it would take is a tiny clip of a pole, and I'd be toast!

One day, I was riding with a friend who flew through the poles without slowing at all. I exclaimed, "How do you ride through without fear of wrecking when you see those two poles?"

He responded sarcastically, "What poles?" When I looked at him in confusion, he explained. "I only see the middle space."

It was all about his focus. While I was looking at the yellow poles and trying to avoid them, he was completely focused on the middle spot between the poles.

Wow, what a difference that bit of knowledge has made. Knowledge and experience are everything. If you focus on either pole, there is a high likelihood of hitting one of the poles and wrecking. That is a proven fact. Why is that? Your brain and eyes will pull the body that way. Once he shared his trick, the fear instantly left me. Now I only focus on the middle space, and I don't even pump my brakes as I sail through. By keeping my focus on the open middle space, I never come close to wrecking by clipping a pole at high speeds.

Let's take a deeper look at some strategies I use to increase my focus.

Strategy 1: Find and Define Your WHY

We've discussed the importance of finding your WHY when you're trying to make a lifestyle change. It's equally important when trying to increase your focus in order to maintain that change. A good way to do this is to become informed. Educate yourself about whatever it is you're trying to do. This will help give you purpose, and purpose is integral to motivation. Your purpose has to supersede the discomfort involved in making the change; if not, the change will likely only be temporary.

Strategy 2: Write It Down

We've all heard about the importance of writing our goals down; it's been said that a dream becomes a goal once it's written down with a date. But neuroscience actually tells us why it's so important to have a plan and write it down. When we write (or even draw) something, we're accessing both external storage and encoding for our brain. External storage basically means you'll remember something much better if you have a visual cue or reminder that you see every day. But the real phenomenon is in the encoding. Mark Murphy, bestselling author and CEO of Leadership IQ, explains how encoding works in his article, "Neuroscience Explains Why You Need to Write Down Your Goals If You Actually Want to Achieve Them":

> Encoding is the biological process by which the things we perceive travel to our brain's hippocampus, where they're analyzed. From there, decisions are made about what gets stored in our long-term memory and, in turn, what gets discarded. Writing improves that encoding process. In other words, when you write it down, it has a much greater chance of being remembered.[47]

---

47 Mark Murphy, "Neuroscience Explains Why You Need To Write Down Your Goals If You Actually Want To Achieve Them," Forbes online magazine, 15 April 2019, *https://www.forbes.com/sites/markmurphy/2018/04/15/neuroscience-explains-why-you-need-to-write-down-your-goals-if-you-actually-want-to-achieve-them/?sh=5dba616e7905.*

Those who write down their goals in vivid detail are 1.2 to 1.4 times more likely to accomplish them. Finalizing your WHY statement and then defining your HOW and WHAT as you write them down is like taking an oath. In fact, if you use my format, including the accountability journaling, you will end up creating a written contract with yourself. You are literally creating a personal promise. The only thing that makes an oath stronger is for you to sign it and have someone you trust and admire sign it as a witness. The Why-How-What Formula is an easy way to do just that and becomes the oath you make with yourself.

Strategy 3: Commit—and Persist

Remember, it takes an average of sixty-six days to modify a negative behavior into a positive quality-of-life behavior.[48] So don't overcommit yourself; I recommend you focus on one change at a time. And remember, there are negative behaviors that will take you even more than sixty-six days to change.

Give your brain time to replace a negative behavior with a positive behavior. It takes patience and focus to make your conscious WHY become your subconscious, automatic, and unthinking WHY.

I encourage you to commit to changing one negative health habit at a time. If you focus on one habit every month, that would be twelve a year. That would be amazingly life-changing! I think a realistic expectation would be to aim for six new

48 Benjamin Gardner, Phillippa Lally, and Jane Wardle, "Making health habitual: the psychology of 'habit-formation' and general practice," US National Library of Medicine and National Institutes of Health, December 2012, *https://www.ncbi.nlm.nih.gov/pmc/articles/PMC3505409/.*

optimal health behaviors per year. Just think: If you could change six negative behaviors into six positive behaviors every year, what would that do for you?

Let's do it today. Commit to change! What's one small decision you could make right now that would take you in the direction you need to go for optimal health? Pull out a piece of paper and brainstorm for a minute. Write down any ideas that come to your mind or that you have learned in this book.

Become Your Own Scientist

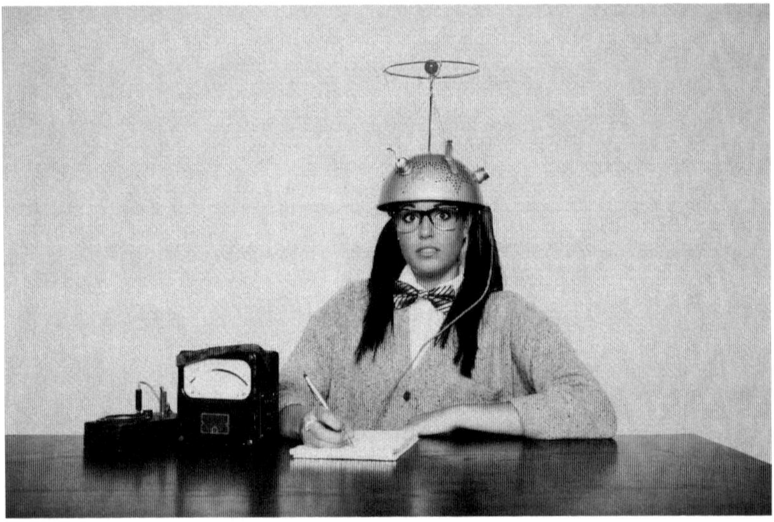

One of the hard lessons I learned over the past few decades is that I have to be my own best health advocate. No doctor is going to do that for me. I have to do the research, become educated, and connect the dots on my own. Essentially, we each have to become our own scientists, and we have to collect data and do the research for our well-being.

While Carla was going to school to be a functional nutritionist, she asked if I would do a daily food-mood-poop journal. She explained that this was an easy way to track data to see if what I ate affected my mood and my poop, which tells us so very much about our overall body health. Because I'm passionate about improving my health, I agreed and started filling out the journal each day.

One day, several weeks into this journaling exercise, I complained to Carla that I had "the runs" and that my stomach was not feeling so good. She immediately went to my journal to see what I had been eating. Lo and behold, she pointed out that, a couple of days earlier, I had stopped for ice cream on my way home from fly fishing. I'd ordered a German chocolate shake, which is my very favorite flavor. She looked at me soberly and said, "Here is the culprit—you cannot have dairy and that much sugar! When you do, you pay a price." I had kept the journal honestly and hadn't hidden anything, and she was right. That shake was the culprit, and we had the data to prove it. Since then, do you think I have had a shake? Absolutely not. The data we have gathered from our science projects has proven so helpful in identifying and eliminating foods that cause me pain.

A good scientist takes meticulous notes. As part of Level 1 in *Eating to Live*, we are going to teach you to become your own scientist and solve your own health dilemmas. We will provide you with easy-to-use templates and meal plans. The Eating to Live Journal will be especially important. Journaling your daily experiences and then answering questions that help you connect the dots in your life will be well worth it. That's how I changed my life! Eliminating all but just one prescription (so far), having my daily pain level drop from an 8 to a 1, and having daily healthy poops (sorry, I know it seems like "too much information," but boy, does this make a difference!) has been life-changing.

One of my favorite expressions is "Is it worth it?" I guarantee that finding your WHY and applying what you learn as you continue to read this book will absolutely be worth it! You'll never perform a more important science experiment than that of determining how to achieve your optimal health so that you can live your best life—and live it for as long as you can.

CHAPTER 3

THE EATING TO LIVE JOURNAL

David Meine

Journaling is absolutely key to the *Eating to Live* program. Journaling is how you will figure out which foods are healthy and helpful for you and which foods your system can't tolerate. By tracking daily food and water intake, pain and discomfort levels, and how well your body is able to discharge waste, you will be able to tell which foods work for you. Tracking this information is integral to healing your gut and to begin accessing levels of health and energy that you may have forgotten were possible.

Daily journaling is pretty simple to do. We have created a form—which you can access as part of Level 1 on the *Eating to Live* website—that you can print and fill out.[49] There is also an *Eating to Live* app for both iOS and Android, available for download through the App Store or Google Play. You are also welcome to create your own journaling system. The important

49 Available at *eatingtolive.com/book/.*

thing is to find a system that works for you so that you can easily track all the necessary information. It's also vital to be completely honest in your reporting. If not, the only person you cheat is yourself.

		EATING TO LIVE JOURNAL	
Time	Daily Activities. Record anything that you think might impact your health positively & negatively.	Record the Foods you Eat How many glasses of water do you drink?	Pain level 1 low- 10 high Dizziness 1- 10 Bowel Movement 1-7. Bloating, Heartburn or Indigestion
7:00 AM			
8:00 AM			
9:00 AM			
10:00 AM			
11:00 AM			
Noon			
1:00 PM			
2:00 PM			
3:00 PM			
4:00 PM			
5:00 PM			
6:00 PM			
7:00 PM			
8:00 PM			
9:00 PM			
10:00 PM			

The form is broken down by the time of day. That doesn't mean you need to write something down for each hour, just when you eat, or if you notice a physical symptom happening at a certain time of day. Here is a breakdown of the items you will need to track in your journal:

- **Daily Activities:** Record anything that you think might impact your health positively or negatively. This would include sleep, exercise, stress, travel, etc.

- **Foods You Eat:** You'll want to write down everything you eat each day. This includes all meals, all snacks... everything! However, this is not like typical "diet" tracking. You don't need to record how much you ate or your calories or carbs or macros. You just need to write down what you eat.
- **Water:** Track the glasses of water you consume throughout the day.
- **Physical Symptoms:** You will rate any pain or dizziness that you have from 1 to 10, track your bowel movements and rate them using the Bristol Stool Chart[50], and record any bloating, heartburn, or indigestion experienced at the time it happens.

In order to gather enough information to draw accurate conclusions, you'll need to journal long enough that you actually start to feel better. For most people, this takes two to four weeks. You will likely begin to notice some patterns in just a few days. If you recognize a food that is causing you any sort of discomfort, remove it immediately from your diet, and continue to track results.

This is where you become the scientist, and tracking all the above items becomes your most important science experiment. You'll start connecting the dots as you are able to identify harmful triggers that upset your particular gut microbiome. As you begin to heal your leaky gut, you'll see pain levels decrease, energy levels increase, and your overall quality of life will start to improve. You'll truly be on your way to achieving your optimal health!

---

50 Find at eatingtolive.com/book/.

CHAPTER 4

THE EATING TO LIVE MEAL PLAN

Carla Meine

"The food you eat can either be the safest and most powerful form of medicine or the slowest form of poison."

—ANN WIGMORE

So back to the question, "What should I eat if I want to be healthy?" Throughout my studies, I've read hundreds of books on nutrition, and most doctors can't even agree on what to eat! Some say that meat is fine, and others say you shouldn't eat any meat. Some say eggs are great for you, while others will say to stay away from eggs. Some say any kind of fruit is great, and others say to eat fruit sparingly and only when in season. Most doctors do seem to agree that fish is wonderful, especially if it's wild-caught and not farmed. But occasionally, I'll find a doctor that says to stay away from all fish.

If the doctors can't agree, how can they expect their patients to be able to figure it out? For years, David and I were living proof of how hard it is. (Remember our years of juicing and the battle with sourdough bread?) It took a lot of experimentation and education to find a meal plan that worked for David to achieve his optimal health, and the answers we got are very individual for him.

Determining the best nutrition lifestyle for each individual takes some trial and error. It takes some time and commitment. It's absolutely true that one person's food can be someone else's poison. It's that individual! The best way to find out what works for you is to start with an elimination diet first, where we will remove certain foods from your diet. Then, as you progress through Levels Two, Three, and Four, you will slowly add some items back in, making sure to journal daily as you go.

To begin, you will remove sugar, gluten, dairy, eggs, poultry, and all meats from your diet. If you've read that sentence and you're now wondering what exactly you *will* eat, that list is longer than you might think. The full list is included in this chapter, but you can eat unlimited vegetables, some fruit (one a day to limit your sugar intake), lots of healthy oils, seafood and fish, non-gluten grains, and even some dark chocolate!

We've also created a meal plan to help you do this. Please note that these meal plans are simply suggestions that include delicious and easy recipes as a way to make Level 1 easier for you. You are welcome to use our recipes or come up with your own. The most important thing is to cook the foods with a healthy oil, like coconut, avocado, or olive. Most people don't get nearly enough healthy oils and fats in their diet, and our recipes are designed to do that. To see some of these yummy recipes, go to https://eatingtolive.com/recipes/. I bet you'll be amazed at how good healthy food can actually taste.

You also have the option to utilize our protein powder and have shakes as a meal replacement. We have created a gluten-free, dairy-free, and sugar-free shake that also tastes good. Our protein powder also has Slendesta as an ingredient, which will help your body to feel full longer and modulate sugars. Even though our protein powder already has 33% of the daily requirement of MCT[51] (medium-chain triglyceride) oil, we encourage you to add a spoonful of MCT oil to your shakes as well. Again, this particular protein powder is not a required part of the program; rather, we offer it as an option to make planning and eating meals easier for you.

The good news about all of this is that you're going to figure out what works for you. You'll be able to determine what your gut needs in order to heal by beginning with a minimal list of foods. Then, once you start feeling better about these foods, you'll start adding foods back. In Level 2, we will teach you very specifically and deliberately how to add eggs and poultry back into your diet and also start supplementation. If you can tolerate that, you'll move to Level 3, where we will carefully reintroduce meats. Level 4 reintroduces dairy. This is the most challenging for people with any form of leaky gut and often comes with bloating, constipation, or diarrhea. In other words, your leaky gut will let you know which foods you tolerate and which you can't.

---

51 Medically reviewed by Dominique Fontaine, BSN, RN, HNB-BC, HWNC, Written by Sharon O'Brien MS, PGDip, "7 Science-Based Benefits of MCT Oil," healthline, 11 November 2020, *https://www.healthline.com/nutrition/mct-oil-benefits.*

Level 1

Vegetables	Peppers*	Fruits	Seafood and Fish	Dairy Substitutes
Arugula	Parsley	Apricots	Clams	Organic, full-fat coconut milk
Artichokes	Radicchio	Apples	Cod	Organic un-sweetened nut milk
Asparagus	Radishes and leaves	Bananas	Crab	Almond milk
Avocado	Romaine lettuce	Blackberries	Halibut	Hazelnut milk
Acorn squash	Rutabaga	Blueberries	Herring	Hemp milk
Beets and beet greens	Scallions	Currants	Lobster	Yogurts made from coconut milk
Bok choy	Shallot	Cranberries	Mackerel	**Non-gluten Grains**
Beans, green	Squash	Cherries	Mussels	Almond four
Broccoli	Sweet potatoes	Dates	Oysters	Other nut flour
Brussel sprouts	Snow peas	Elderberries	Salmon	Amaranth
Bamboo shoots	Spinach	Figs	Sardines	Arrowroot
Chard	Seaweed	Grapes	Sea bass	Coconut flour
Chicory	Sea vegetable	Grapefruit	Shrimp	Cassava flour
Cilantro	Turnips and turnip greens	Goji berries	Trout	Flaxseeds/ flax
Collard greens	Tomatoes*	Honeydew melon	Tuna	Sorghum
Cabbage	Watercress	Kiwi	**Oils (cold-pressed)**	Tapioca

Celery	Water chestnuts	Lemon	Avocado oil	**Noodles**
Cucumber	Zucchini	Limes	Flax oil	Cappello's fettuccine
Carrots	Yams	Mango	Hemp oil	Pasta slim
Cauliflower	White potato (limit 1 per week)	Oranges	Olive oil (extra virgin)	Shirataki noodles
Chives	**Flavorings**	Pineapple	Nut oil	Kelp noodles
Dandelion greens	Coconut aminos	Pumpkin	MCT oil	Miracle noodles & Kanten pasta
Eggplant*	Herbs and spices	Pears	**Cooking Oils**	Miracle rice
Endive	Horseradish	Papaya	Avocado oil	Sweet potato noodles
Escarole	Himalayan sea salt	Peaches	Clarified butter/Ghee	Spaghetti squash noodles
Green peas (Green, split peas, black-eyed peas)	Mustard	Plums	Coconut oil	Zucchini and squash noodles
Garlic	Nutritional yeast	Pomegran-ates	Pecan oil	**Bone Broth**
Hearts of palm	Pickles	Passion fruit	Sesame oil	1 cup per day, gluten-free, organic
Kale	Sauerkraut	Prunes	**Sweeteners** (1 tsp. per day)	**Beverages**
Lettuce (all but iceberg)	Sea salt (preferably iodized)	Raspberries	Honey	Water
Leeks	Tamari (gluten-free only)	Rhubarb	Just Like Sugar	Club soda
Mushrooms	Wasabi (gluten-free only)	Raisins	Real maple syrup	Coffee (limit 2 cups per day)

Mustard greens		Strawberries	Molasses	Tea (black, green, white, red root, oolong, match, herbal)
Mizuna		Tangerines	Monk fruit	Yerba mate
Onions		Watermelon	Sorghum	Kombucha tea
Okra		**Vinegars**	Stevia	**Chocolate**
Olives		Any, if no added sugar	Swerve	70% or greater, 1 oz. per day
			Xylitol	

**unless you have issues*

Notes about Foods in Level 1

- Eat lots of greens (this one shouldn't surprise any of us).
- Fill up on salads full of mixed greens, spinach, avocado, artichokes, asparagus, carrots, etc.
- Use olive oil-based dressings without sugar where possible.
- Try to eat wild-caught fish, as farmed fish is usually fed corn and soy.
- Have a cup of organic, gluten-free bone broth every day. Bone broth delivers multiple health benefits without the adverse effects of meat; it's high in nutritional value, has collagen that is good for joints and skin, helps reduce inflammation, and helps heal leaky gut, just to name a few. For additional information on the benefits of bone broth, as well as my favorite bone broth recipe, see our blog post at: *https://eatingtolive.com/bone-broth/*.

When it comes to considering making changes to your current diet, please ask yourself, "Is what you're doing working?" If not, why not give this a try? We've learned through personal experience that not only is it doable, it's absolutely life-changing. Once you remember how good it feels to *feel good*, you'll never want to go back!

CHAPTER 5

DRINK MORE WATER

Carla Meine

How much water have you had to drink today?

If you're like the great majority of my clients, you haven't had nearly enough. I find it fascinating that most people say they know how important water is for their health, yet most of them aren't drinking even close to the amount they need to be healthy. When I ask a client how much water they think they should be drinking, most of them can tell me they should drink half their weight in ounces of water each day.

That means if you are a 150-pound woman, you should consume seventy-five ounces of water a day. That's not necessarily an accurate amount, by the way, as the amount of water you need is based on more than just your weight (we'll talk about this more below). But I rarely find a person who's actually consuming that much water on a daily basis. Some clients tell me they drink less than twenty ounces of water a day. Or they say they're drinking plenty of water because they count coffee, soda, juices, etc., toward their daily intake. Unfortunately, only pure, filtered water counts toward your daily water goal.

It's hard to overstate the importance of water when it comes to healthy living. As a Certified Functional Nutrition Counselor, water intake is just as important as food intake analysis as we work toward solving health issues and achieving optimal health. It's been said that water is the most important nutrient we put into our bodies. We can live three weeks without food, but we can't go more than three days without water. Our bodies are made up of 45%–60% water, depending on age, gender, and weight (babies are more like 80%). Every organ and tissue in the body is made up of a majority of water. Your lungs are around 80% water, your brain is over 80% water, your muscles and heart are over 75% water, your skin is over 70% water[52]—I could go on, but you get the idea. Water is critical to your survival.

Many of my clients worry that if they drink more water, they'll have to go to the bathroom more often. This is a valid concern, as urinary incontinence affects about 17.5 million women in the US[53] and is a problem that can really disrupt your life. I've assembled a lot of helpful information about why this is—and what you can do about it—in a post on our website.[54] If

---

52 Medically reviewed by Jillian Kubala, MS, RD, Written by Claire Sissons, "Where is water in the body, subheader — What is the average percentage of water in the human body?" Medical News Today, 27 May 2020, *https://www.medicalnewstoday.com/articles/what-percentage-of-the-human-body-is-water#where-in-the-body.*

53 Andrea Nakayama, Urinary Intensive, June-July 2020.

54 You can access this post (and many other informational posts) at *eatingtolive.com/book/.*

this is something you or someone you love struggles with, I encourage you to research it further.

For our purposes here, just know that water intake doesn't affect incontinence the way you might think it does. For example, if you're drinking too little water, it causes your urine to be highly concentrated, which can irritate the bladder mucosa and lead to incontinence. Also, it's interesting to note that urinary incontinence is one of the major risk factors for falling among elderly populations. This is because dehydration often causes brain fog/confusion and balance issues, and incontinence causes people to restrict fluid intake because they fear incontinence; it's a vicious cycle that could actually be helped by proper treatment for urinary incontinence and through increasing water consumption.

Drinking water is an important part of your body's daily detoxification process. If you don't drink enough water, it can cause some serious urinary problems down the road. And, if you're drinking beverages that act as diuretics (coffee, tea, soda, energy drinks, and alcohol—caffeine and alcohol are the worst offenders here[55]), you're exacerbating the problem. Additionally, beverages with high sugar content, such as fruit juices, keep the body from absorbing the water it needs.[56] The bottom line? Instead of choosing those caffeine- or sugar-filled drinks, reach for a refreshing glass of water.

Let's take a look at how water affects specific parts of your body:

---

55 Andrea Nakayama, Urinary Intensive, June-July 2020.

56 Madison Conley, "3 kinds of drinks that actually dehydrate you — and why," Insider, 19 October 2018, *https://www.insider.com/drinks-that-cause-dehydration-2018-10.*

Digestive Tract

A simple example of the importance of water is found in the digestive tract. If you don't drink enough water, the body will compensate by pulling water from your stools, leaving your colon dry. The result of that is constipation. When I'm dealing with clients that are constipated, my first question is, "How much water do you drink?" Rarely are they drinking enough. When they increase their water intake, constipation starts to go away. We usually have some food issues we need to resolve for constipation to completely go away, but water is a really simple solution to start with.

Detox Organs

Another good example is detoxification. Through my education, I've learned so much about the liver and the kidneys and the immensely important role they play in detoxing the body. Your body has to have enough water to help move waste products and toxins out of the body. If you're not hydrated enough, then the body can't do that properly.

Do you know anyone that suffers from urinary tract infections (UTIs) or kidney stones on a regular basis? You probably do; more women go to the doctor for urinary tract infections than almost anything else.[57] A UTI is essentially inflammation of the urinary bladder and/or the urethra, and women are especially susceptible to these simply due to our anatomy. If you are prone to these infections or to kidney stones, you should increase your water intake. It might not be the only solution, but it's a pretty easy one to try to see if it helps. Those who trade in soda for water often see a big improvement in this area.

---

57 Andrea Nakayama, Urinary Intensive, June-July 2020.

Skin

Did you know it's often visibly obvious that you're dehydrated? Your skin gives it away. You can have more skin disorders and wrinkles when you're not taking in a sufficient amount of water on a regular basis. Let's do a simple experiment: Make a goal for thirty days to drink plenty of water. Maybe even cut out some of the diuretic beverages you're consuming. Be sure to take a "before" and "after" picture of your skin and see if it doesn't look healthier at the end of the thirty days. My prediction is that if you're not currently hydrating adequately, you'll see a difference—and so will others.

Muscles

The first area where I notice dehydration in my body is in my muscles. If I haven't consumed enough water in a day, I almost always get leg cramps at night. I increased my potassium intake, and that helped, but if I don't consume enough water, the cramps still happen. Since the muscles are made up of so much water, keeping them hydrated enables them to work harder and longer and assists in building additional muscles. Drinking the right amount of water is important in any type of athletics and has a positive effect on performance.

Electrolytes

Another thing that helps with hydration and muscle recovery is electrolytes. Electrolytes are essential minerals in our bodies (think sodium, calcium, and potassium) that are vital for many key bodily functions. Electrolyte balance is intricately tied to the health of our urinary systems. We lose electrolytes as we sweat, which is why you hear about them in association with working out and in ads for sports drinks. We also lose electrolytes if we have a fever, diarrhea, or are often vomiting.

Basically, anything that disturbs water balance is also going to disturb electrolyte balance.

Sweat is how our bodies help regulate our systems and cool us down when we're overheated. It's an important bodily function, but it's also how we lose a lot of electrolytes. When you exercise, drink more water than you think you need to. I instruct endurance athletes to drink every fifteen minutes, whether they're thirsty or not. By the time you feel thirsty, dehydration is already in process. Dehydration in any form and electrolyte imbalance cause a big decrease in performance. Staying on a water-drinking schedule is the easiest way to avoid any of these issues and to keep your body performing at its very best.

Some other benefits of drinking water:[58]

- Water helps oxygenate the body. Blood is more than 90% water, and your blood carries oxygen to various parts of your body.
- It lubricates your joints. Cartilage is 80% water, and when you're dehydrated, your joints lose their shock-absorption ability, which equals joint pain.
- Hydration helps your brain. Staying hydrated cushions the brain, spinal cord, and other sensitive tissues. Water is also involved in hormone and neurotransmitter production, which means prolonged dehydration actually interferes with your ability to think and reason.

---

58 Medically reviewed by Karen Cross, FNP, MSN, Written by James McIntosh, "Fifteen benefits of drinking water," Medical News Today, 16 July 2018, *https://www.medicalnewstoday.com/articles/290814.*

- Water affects your blood pressure. When you don't get enough water, your blood can become thicker, which increases your blood pressure.
- Staying hydrated prevents dry mouth, which is actually more important than you might realize. Saliva enables digestion. It also keeps your mouth, nose, and eyes moist, which prevents friction and damage. Drinking water also helps keep your mouth clean and can reduce tooth decay.

Water and Weight Loss

If you've ever tried to lose weight, you probably know that most weight loss regimens include upping your water intake. That's because hydration is key for many factors that assist in weight loss. We've already touched on some of those things, like the importance of waste removal and body detoxing, for which water is integral. But water also works as a natural appetite suppressant. Water helps your body feel full and reduces those feelings of hunger. Also, you might think you're hungry when, in actuality, your body just needs some water. If you reach for water before food, it might reduce extra snacking.

Additionally, research says that drinking water helps burn calories. Resting energy expenditure increases by 24%–30% for at least sixty minutes after drinking water.[59] Water is literally a pure source of energy! Water is also necessary to burn fat. The first step of metabolizing fat is hydrolysis, which happens when water molecules interact with triglycerides (in

---

59 Adda Bjarnadottir, MS, RDN (Ice), "How Drinking More Water Can Help You Lose Weight," Healthline, 14, December 2020, *https://www.healthline.com/nutrition/drinking-water-helps-with-weight-loss.*

other words, fats) to create glycerol and fatty acids.[60] Drinking enough water helps burn fat consumed through food and drink as well as stored fat.

So, how much water should you drink?

Just like there is no one-size-fits-all answer as far as dietary recommendations go, there really is no standard answer for how much water to drink. The amount you require depends on a variety of factors, including:

- Age
- Body size
- Activity level
- Diet
- Where you live (humidity, sun exposure, temperature, altitude, etc.)
- Health status

It's also important to remember that, as you have water coming in, you also have water going out through your skin, lungs, and GI tract (urine and stools).

As a baseline, take a look at what the US National Academies of Sciences, Engineering, and Medicine recommends. They say that for the average, healthy adult living in a temperate climate, getting adequate daily fluid means:

---

60 Medically reviewed by Elaine K. Luo, M.D., Written by Jennifer Huizen, "Getting enough water, subheader — Can water help you lose weight?" Medical News Today, 28 June 2018, *https://www.medicalnewstoday.com/articles/322296#getting-enough-water.*

- About 15.5 cups (3.7 liters) of fluids a day for men
- About 11.5 cups (2.7 liters) of fluids a day for women[61]

I say that's a good starting point. Then, through paying attention and journaling your experience, you will be able to determine if that is actually enough water for your body. Based both on available research and my own experience with clients, chances are you're not drinking nearly enough.

I don't think it's possible to overstate how important water consumption is in order for you to function properly every day. It should be an absolute must for you each day. If this is something that is extra hard, make it a game. Something that works for me is to have a 24-ounce container that I fill with water at least four times per day. I see if I can drink one by a certain time, and then I fill it up again. Once I've had all my water for the day, I tell myself I can have another beverage if I'm still thirsty. Most days, I find I am completely content to just drink water. It really is a pretty amazing cure-all. Whether you're tired, hungry, have a headache, or just need a pick-me-up, a glass of water—or two—might be all you need.

---

61 Mayo Clinic Staff, "How much water do you need?" Mayo Clinic, 14 October 2020, *https://www.mayoclinic.org/healthy-lifestyle/nutrition-and-healthy-eating/in-depth/water/art-20044256#.*

WHY I GAVE UP GLUTEN: MY PSORIASIS-FREE LIFE

Kristie Frost

Over the past year or so, I started having problems with my skin. I'd never had anything like it before, and I think it might have been triggered by the onset of menopause. I first noticed it on my left elbow when this weird, oblong-shaped, dry patch of skin appeared. I kept putting various lotions and creams on it, but it didn't help. It quickly became really crusty and flaky, but worst of all, it was incredibly itchy.

This was different than any dry skin I'd experienced before. The itch felt like a fire burning underneath my skin. And every time I scratched, it burned more. I thought it might be really bad eczema, so I kept putting cream on, but nothing helped.

Next, I noticed a dime-sized patch on my other elbow as well. Was this happening because of how I placed my elbows on my counter at work, I wondered? Then I went camping with my family, and the back of my neck became itchy. I thought I must've had a tick and asked my husband to look at it. "No," he said, "It's just a really red, dry patch—kind of like your elbow." My problem was obviously spreading, and I was so itchy I was starting to lose my mind! Plus, it was embarrassing. I was constantly scratching myself as if I had cooties.

Around this time, Carla came in for her nail appointment. I've been doing her nails for about thirty years, and we've become good friends. I shared my psoriasis woes with her. "Oh, Kristie," she said, "I'll bet that gluten is causing that. Your body just can't tolerate it. You've got to give up wheat and gluten. I know it will make a huge difference!" What? Give up bread? Pizza? Pastries? I didn't want to believe that could be the answer, but I started wondering if it could be true.

I happened to see something on TV where Kim Kardashian talked about a skin condition she had called psoriasis. I Googled it and read that the most common areas affected were elbows, knees, hands, and the back of the neck. This had to be what I had!

I kept Googling and found an account on Instagram about naturally reversing skin conditions like psoriasis. He made a connection between psoriasis and wheat/gluten consumption. I remembered what Carla had said, and I started to pay attention to how I felt when I ate anything with wheat or gluten, and I noticed I felt overfull, a little bloated, even when I hadn't eaten that much. I decided to reduce the amount of wheat I was eating. I wasn't super strict, but I tried to eliminate breads or processed foods that contained wheat. I noticed I felt better, but my psoriasis remained.

I went to the dermatologist, who prescribed me some special cream. By this time, I had a particularly bad spot on my hand in a patch by my thumb. It seemed especially hyperactive, probably due to how often I wash my hands as a nail artist. I mentioned my thoughts about the wheat connection, but he was adamant. "Nope, it has nothing to do with the way you eat. Don't worry about it!" he insisted. The cream he gave me was a harsh steroid that could only be used for fourteen days.

I decided not to eat any wheat at all from Halloween until Thanksgiving. During this time, I also used the steroid cream the doctor gave me. By mid-November, the big patch on my elbow was completely gone. It looked like fresh skin! The patches on my other elbow, neck, and even my hand were all pretty much cleared up as well. Then, Thanksgiving hit.

I didn't go crazy, but I ate the mashed potatoes and the rolls and the pie. The very next day, I had a dime-sized patch on my left elbow, my other elbow was beet red, and I was itchy again. I felt like the evidence was undeniable—what I had eaten had caused the psoriasis to come back!

Now I was really committed and went off all wheat and gluten. I was very strict about it for three weeks. I used the steroid cream for a few days, and everything cleared up. Then... Christmas. I come from a big, Greek family. We take our food seriously! We use lots of filo dough and make delicious pastries, and food is one of our love languages. For us, the holidays mean homemade baklava and spanakopita. I always make a delicious horiatiki salad with homemade croutons. I decided that I didn't care what I ate and enjoyed it all.

By New Year's Eve, I was toast. I was a complete, itchy mess. In addition to the usual spots, the entire back of my neck was covered, there were spots on both ears, and my elbows were worse. Plus, instead of the patch on my thumb, the whole palm of my hand was inflamed. It was growing! This wasn't a small reaction. This was a terrible price to pay for some pastry!

It was obvious I had to cut out wheat entirely, and since then, I have. Here's the formula that works for me: When I avoid wheat and gluten, I don't suffer from psoriasis. I'm feeling additional benefits as well. I no longer have stomach bloating issues or feel sick and overfull after eating. I'm more regular in the bathroom. I've dropped a few pounds and hope to drop a few more. Overall, I just feel better!

Giving up foods I truly enjoy has not been easy. But every time I slip even a little bit—if I even tear off a piece of my son's tortilla when we go out for Mexican food—my elbows go red, and I start to itch. I miss cookies. I miss pizza! And I don't know how the next big family holiday (Easter) is going to play out. But here is what I do know: When I eat those things, I pay. My skin communicates the message loud and clear.

It takes a strong WHY to remain committed despite food temptations. So what's my WHY? I want to live a pain-free, itch-free life without ugly, red blotches on my skin. I choose to do what it takes to live without psoriasis. In my experience, psoriasis isn't curable, but it is controllable. I choose control. It might not be easy, but it's definitely worth it!

LEVEL 2

CHAPTER 1

AN INTRODUCTION TO LEVEL 2

Carla Meine

Advancing to Level 2 means that you have successfully eliminated the foods required in Level One and tracked all your results over the past few weeks. Take a moment to think about how you are feeling as you begin Level 1. How are your energy levels compared to before you started this journey? How are you sleeping? What are your pain levels like? You might want to journal some of your overall thoughts about how you feel as you begin this next level in *Eating to Live*.

In this level, we will address some additional crucial components of living a healthy life: healthy sleep and avoiding NSAIDs. Both are key building blocks of health and very necessary as you continue healing your gut and regaining energy and a sense of well-being on this journey.

The Level 2 food additions are pretty simple. It includes everything from Level 1, plus poultry, eggs, nuts, seeds, and rice. Here is the Level 2 food chart with the new food categories included:

Level 2

Vegetables	Peppers*	**Fruits**	**Seafood and Fish**	**Dairy Substitutes**
Arugula	Parsley	Apricots	Clams	Organic, full-fat coconut milk
Artichokes	Radicchio	Apples	Cod	Organic unsweetened nut milk
Asparagus	Radishes and leaves	Bananas	Crab	Almond milk
Avocado	Romaine lettuce	Blackberries	Halibut	Hazelnut milk
Acorn squash	Rutabaga	Blueberries	Herring	Hemp milk
Beets and beet greens	Scallions	Currants	Lobster	Yogurts made from coconut milk
Bok choy	Shallot	Cranberries	Mackerel	**Non-gluten Grains**
Beans, green	Squash	Cherries	Mussels	Almond four
Broccoli	Sweet potatoes	Dates	Oysters	Other nut flour
Brussel sprouts	Snow peas	Elderberries	Salmon	Amaranth
Bamboo shoots	Spinach	Figs	Sardines	Arrowroot
Chard	Seaweed	Grapes	Sea bass	Coconut flour
Chicory	Sea vegetable	Grapefruit	Shrimp	Cassava flour
Cilantro	Turnips and turnip greens	Goji berries	Trout	Flaxseeds/ flax

Collard greens	Tomatoes*	Honeydew melon	Tuna	Sorghum
Cabbage	Watercress	Kiwi	**Oils (cold-pressed)**	Tapioca
Celery	Water chestnuts	Lemon	Avocado oil	**Noodles**
Cucumber	Zucchini	Limes	Flax oil	Cappello's fettuccine
Carrots	Yams	Mango	Hemp oil	Pasta slim
Cauliflower	White potato (limit 1 per week)	Oranges	Olive oil (extra virgin)	Shirataki noodles
Chives	**Flavorings**	Pineapple	Nut oil	Kelp noodles
Dandelion greens	Coconut aminos	Pumpkin	MCT oil	Miracle noodles & Kanten pasta
Eggplant*	Herbs and spices	Pears	**Cooking Oils**	Miracle rice
Endive	Horseradish	Papaya	Avocado oil	Sweet potato noodles
Escarole	Himalayan sea salt	Peaches	Clarified butter/Ghee	Spaghetti squash noodles
Green peas (Green, split peas, black-eyed peas)	Mustard	Plums	Coconut oil	Zucchini and squash noodles
Garlic	Nutritional yeast	Pomegranates	Pecan oil	Rice
Hearts of palm	Pickles	Passion fruit	Sesame oil	Bone Broth
Kale	Sauerkraut	Prunes	**Sweeteners (1 tsp. per day)**	1 cup per day, gluten-free, organic
Lettuce (all but iceberg)	Sea salt (preferably iodized)	Raspberries	Honey	Beverages
Leeks	Tamari (gluten-free only)	Rhubarb	Just Like Sugar	Water

Mushrooms	Wasabi (gluten-free only)	Raisins	Real maple syrup	Club soda
Mustard greens		Strawberries	Molasses	Coffee (limit 2 cups per day)
Mizuna		Tangerines	Monk fruit	Tea (black, green, white, red root, oolong, match, herbal)
Onions		Watermelon	Sorghum	Yerba mate
Okra		**Vinegars**	Stevia	Kombucha tea
Olives		Any, if no added sugar	Swerve	**Chocolate**
			Xylitol	70% or greater, 1 oz. per day
Poultry**	**Eggs**** (pasture-raised only)	**Nuts & Seeds**** (if you can tolerate them)		
Chicken	Chicken	Tree Nuts • Almonds • Walnuts • Hazelnuts • Cashews • Brazil nuts • Pistachios • Macadamia nuts • Pecans • Chestnuts • Pinenuts		

Duck	Duck	Seeds • Sunflower • Pumpkin • Sesame • Flax • Chia • Psyllium		
Dove		Peanuts		
Goose		Tahini		
Pheasant		Sunflower butter		
Turkey		Almond butter		

**unless you have issues*
***Level 2 food group additions*

We recommend limiting poultry to four to six ounces for women and six to ten ounces for men per day, depending on your size. When buying poultry, be sure to look for pasture-raised. This is important because pasture-raised will contain more natural omega-3s and vitamin D, as they are outdoors more and can forage naturally for food. (This is why grandma's chickens and eggs were the best—they are both healthier and taste better!)

If you can't find pasture-raised, then free-range and hormone-free are the next best thing. Unfortunately, a chicken labeled "free-range" simply means it had access to a tiny door that leads to a tiny outdoor space for five minutes per day. It doesn't mean they actually spent five minutes out there. Labels are misleading at best, so be careful. The most important thing is to not get the extra hormones contained in many poultry products, so be diligent when picking them.

Just like in Level 1, it's best to eat vegetables that are organic, and wild-caught fish and seafood.

Nuts and Seeds

One of the exciting things you may be looking forward to in Level 2 is adding nuts and seeds to your meal plan. As we've already discussed, please make sure that you add them one at a time and then wait three days to watch for any increased pain, bloating, indigestion, gas, or bowel movement changes. For example, if you add almonds to your meal plan today, don't add any other new foods for at least three days. That way, you will know that any unusual changes are due to the almonds and not something else. If, after three days, you are still feeling great, then you can add some sunflower seeds or another type of nut or seed, repeating the process.

Although they are considered to be a healthy food, nuts and seeds are challenging for many people. It's critical to pay close attention to the signs your body gives you as you add them back into your diet, one at a time.

Even though David loves nuts and seeds, there are only a few of them that he can have without experiencing pain. One of the hardest things to accept is when foods you love, that are supposedly healthy, are harming your body. And, because everyone is so unique, only you can figure out what those foods are for your body. That's why we always talk about you being the scientist, and your body the lab experiment.

Rice

Like nuts and seeds, rice can be a problematic food for some people. David notices that he can have a little rice, but if he eats too much, he will have bloating and pain. Like most of his challenging foods, he finds it easier to just stay away from it rather than moderate it.

You may be different. You may find when you have white rice you have no issues, but brown rice causes you indigestion and gas—or vice versa. This is why you need to make sure you only add one type of rice at a time, and then wait, watch, and journal the results.

You will probably need to spend several weeks in Level 2. Each time you add a new food—poultry, eggs, nuts, seeds, and rice (including different types of each of these food categories)—you need to wait three days between each one. Each new food needs to be thoroughly vetted for your body. It takes a while to determine if any of these foods are causing you problems, but ultimately, it is time well spent as you work toward healing your gut.

On the *Eating to Live* website, you can access the Level 2 meal plan along with many Level 2 recipes. Some will have poultry and eggs in them. Others will be additional Level 2 recipes. You are free to continue using any recipes from Level 1 as well. You can also always add your favorite vegetable dishes. Just make sure they are cooked with good oils, like coconut, avocado, or olive oil. Also, as we did in Level 1, we only use natural spices and ingredients so that we keep potential food sensitivities to a minimum.

The goal is to still eat gluten-free, sugar-free, and dairy-free. We won't add other meats until Level 3.

Make sure you continue to track everything in your Eating to Live Journal daily. What did you eat? How are you feeling? How are your bowel movements? Are you having any gas, bloating, pain, or nausea? What about skin issues like acne, eczema, psoriasis, or Pityriasis Rosea? If so, are they getting better or worse as you remove certain foods from your diet?

As you track, you will begin to connect the dots. *You* are the scientist, and your body is the lab experiment. Only you can figure out what foods your body really needs and which ones you need to avoid. Don't worry—the more you do this, the easier it will become. Stick with it! If you do, you will ultimately find your way to optimal health.

When diet is wrong, medicine is of no use. When diet is correct, medicine is of no need.

—AYURVEDIC PROVERB

CHAPTER 2

GET PLENTY OF SLEEP

David Meine

Scientists have discovered a revolutionary new treatment that makes you live longer. It enhances your memory and makes you more creative. It makes you look more attractive. It keeps you slim and lowers food cravings. It protects you from cancer and dementia. It wards off colds and the flu. It lowers your risk of heart attacks and stroke, not to mention diabetes. You'll even feel happier, less depressed, and less anxious. Are you interested?

—DR. MATTHEW WALKER, WHY WE SLEEP, P. 107

The above "advertisement" is not referencing a too-good-to-be-true health elixir. It's not an exaggeration. It is a scientifically-based description of the amazing whole-body benefits of sleep. The power of consistent and sufficient good sleep would be difficult to exaggerate. In fact, the more I learn about it, the more I'm convinced that sleep truly is *the* key to good health. But the sad truth is, hardly anyone gets the amount or quality they need of this life-sustaining and life-saving commodity.

Many people don't prioritize sleep. These are the folks who consistently "burn the candle at both ends," trying to fit "just one more thing" into their day. A friend recently said to me, referring to this candle-burning analogy, "I'm not even a candle anymore! I'm just a ball of wax!" This has actually become a lifestyle we laud here in the US, all the while watching our health and quality of life decline. There are also situations where life circumstances prohibit sleep, such as my friend with a type 1-diabetic son whose health needs constantly interrupt their sleep. New parents or people who are on-call for work 24/7 might also relate to longing for better and more sleep.

However, studies show that even more people don't get adequate sleep, or they get very low-quality, interrupted sleep, because they actually lack the ability to sleep, even though they give themselves adequate opportunity to do so. Insomnia has become an increasingly rampant and widespread problem. It's estimated that one of every nine people (or 40 million Americans) meets the strict clinical criteria for an insomnia diagnosis.[62] But the experts estimate that insomnia is much more prevalent than that, with two of every three people having regular difficulty with falling or staying asleep every night.

Dr. Matthew Walker, the director of the Center for Human Sleep Science and the author of the book *Why We Sleep*, puts it this way:

---

62 "3 Extent and Health Consequences of Chronic Sleep Loss and Sleep Disorders, excerpt from Sleep Disorders and Sleep Deprivation: An Unmet Public Health Problem" The National Academies, 2006, *https://www.ncbi.nlm.nih.gov/books/NBK19961/.*

> Without belaboring the point, insomnia is one of the most pressing and prevalent medical issues facing modern society, yet few speak of it this way, recognize the burden, or feel there is a need to act. That the "sleep aid" industry, encompassing prescription sleeping medications and over-the-counter sleep remedies, is worth an astonishing $30 billion a year in the US is perhaps the only statistic one needs in order to realize how truly grave the problem is. Desperate millions of us are willing to pay a lot of money for a good night's sleep.[63]

In actuality, less than one-third of all adults in all developed nations get the recommended (necessary!) eight hours of sleep each night. In 2018, the World Health Organization (WHO) declared sleep loss an epidemic throughout all industrialized nations.[64]

Walker continues:

> I was once fond of saying, "Sleep is the third pillar of good health, alongside diet and exercise." I have changed my tune. Sleep is more than a pillar; it is the foundation on which the other two health bastions sit. Take away the bedrock of sleep, or weaken it just a little, and careful eating or physical exercise become less than effective.... Every major system, tissue, and organ of your body suffers when sleep becomes short.[65]

---

63 Matthew Walker, *Why We Sleep: Unlocking the Power of Sleep and Dreams*, (Scribner; 1st edition, October 1, 2017), p. 243.

64 *Sleepless in America,* National Geographic, *https://youtu.be/1qlxKFEE7Ec.*

65 Matthew Walker, *Why We Sleep: Unlocking the Power of Sleep and Dreams*, (Scribner; 1st edition, October 1, 2017), p. 164.

We've already discussed my personal battle with sleep apnea, and I've shared the life-changing result of treating that condition. But let's take a deeper look at why sleep is so very integral to every part of our health and wellness. Much of what I've learned comes from Walker's best-selling book, mentioned above. I highly encourage you to read it from cover to cover, especially if you are one of the millions of us who think that getting six to seven hours or less of sleep a night is okay. Scientific studies make it undeniably clear that "the shorter your sleep, the shorter your lifespan." Let's take a look at how sleep relates to a number of issues we've discussed in this book.

Sleep and Aging

As young adults, we often "burn the candle at both ends" through our college years and work crazy hours getting established in our profession. Then we spend our twenties and thirties caring for young children who often interrupt our sleep. By the time all that has settled down in our midlife and into older age and we have more time to sleep, a lot of us simply *can't* sleep. Now that we finally have the opportunity (and the wisdom!) to get a full night of restorative sleep, our bodies simply don't let us! It seems the cruelest of Mother Nature's tricks.

Science affirms that the older we get, the more problematic sleep gets. This may be a side effect of medications we take as we age. It can also be a side effect of other things, such as menopause. Women who are premenopausal may find themselves struggling to be able to sleep fairly regularly. And by the time they are post-menopausal, most women feel less satisfied with their sleep, with 61% of women that age reporting full insomnia symptoms.[66] Sleep apnea is another widespread culprit. The average age of someone diagnosed with sleep apnea is fifty.[67]

One sleep myth that persists is that older people require less sleep. This claim, however, is false. Studies show that older adults need as much sleep as younger adults, but they are far worse at getting it. Also frightening is the fact that many older adults do not connect their lack of quality sleep with the deterioration in their health. Seniors often visit their doctor for help with their health issues, but rarely ask about their sleep issues.

Of course, not all medical issues that accompany aging are due to lack of sleep. But, according to the experts, far more of our age-related ailments are related to sleep impairment than most people (including many doctors) realize. Consider the following information, based on multiple epidemiologic sleep studies conducted among elderly adults:

> Inefficient sleep is no small thing, as studies assessing tens of thousands of older adults show. Even when controlling for factors such as body mass index, gender, race, history of smoking, frequency of exercise, and medications, the lower an older individual's sleep efficiency score, the higher their mortality risk, the worse their physical health, the more likely they are

66 Medically Reviewed by Dr. Ealena Callender, Written by Danielle Pacheco, "Menopause and Sleep," Sleep Foundation, 22 January 2021, *https://www.sleepfoundation.org/articles/menopause-and-sleep.*

67 American Technion Society, "Twenty Somethings with Sleep Apnea Most Likely to Die," Newswise, 23 February 2005, *https://www.newswise.com/articles/twenty-somethings-with-sleep-apnea-most-likely-to-die.*

> to suffer from depression, the less energy they report, and the lower their cognitive function, typified by forgetfulness. Any individual, no matter what age, will exhibit physical ailments, mental health instability, reduced alertness, and impaired memory if their sleep is chronically disrupted. The problem in aging is that family members observe these daytime features in older relatives and jump to a diagnosis of dementia, overlooking the possibility that bad sleep is an equally likely cause.[68]

If you are an older adult and struggling to be able to get enough quality sleep, please don't seek a sleep aid prescription. Instead, find a board-certified sleep medicine provider who can help you with many scientifically proven, non-pharmacological solutions for sleep.

Sleep and Your Brain

Entire books have been written about how sleep affects memory. Good sleep is one of the most powerful learning aids available, and we can boost our brain's retention abilities exponentially if we sleep both before and after learning. Conversely, even a small lack of sleep impairs your ability to learn and your ability to retain information. It even affects your baseline IQ. Sleep deprivation affects your ability to perform well—so much so that world-class athletes consciously choose to nap before important games and races.

---

68 Matthew Walker, *Why We Sleep: Unlocking the Power of Sleep and Dreams*, (Scribner; 1st edition, October 1, 2017), p. 97.

Lack of sleep affects motor skills and impulse control on a life-threatening level. People who are awake for nineteen hours test at the same level of cognitive impairment as people who are legally drunk. If you get less than five hours of sleep, you have three times the chance of crashing your car if you drive. More accidents are caused by drowsy driving than drunk driving—in the US, that's over 250,000 every day![69] None of this is helped by the fact that we are pretty bad at assessing our own impairment levels and consistently underestimate levels of sleep deprivation. Chances are, we're probably more adversely affected by it than we think.

Sleep and Alzheimer's

If you're anything like me, you have a true fear of developing Alzheimer's later in life. This fear is justified—Alzheimer's is not a normal part of aging. It is a devastating disease that has become one of the largest public health challenges (not to mention economic challenges) of the twenty-first century. In the US, someone develops Alzheimer's every sixty-five seconds. One out of every ten adults over sixty-five years old has Alzheimer's.[70] That's over 40 million people!

Sleep disturbance may actually be an early warning sign of Alzheimer's or contribute to it. Insufficient sleep is now being recognized as a key lifestyle factor that determines whether or not you will develop the disease. In fact, sleep experts are

---

69 "Acute Sleep Deprivation and Crash Risk," Foundation for Traffic Safety, December 2016, *https://www.aaafoundation.org/acute-sleep-deprivation-and-crash-risk.*

70 "The Alzheimer's Disease Crisis - By the Numbers," USA Against Alzheimers, 2021, *https://www.usagainstalzheimers.org/learn/alzheimers-crisis.*

now saying that getting too little sleep in your adult years will significantly raise your risk of developing Alzheimer's.

If that's true, however, the converse should also be true. Sleep scientists are now conducting studies showing strong evidence that, by improving our sleep, we also reduce our risk of developing Alzheimer's, or at least delay its onset. In studies where middle-aged and older adults have had their sleep disorders successfully treated, "their rate of cognitive decline slowed significantly, and further delayed the onset of Alzheimer's disease by five to ten years."[71]

Obviously, insufficient sleep is not the only risk factor associated with Alzheimer's disease. However, it is clear that prioritizing sleep is an incredibly important factor for lowering our risk. This fact alone should be motivation for all of us to prioritize getting better sleep throughout our adult life.

Sleep and Your Immune System

It should come as no surprise that sleep and our immune systems are closely linked. What might surprise you is how much a good night's sleep improves our immune system's ability to defend us. This applies to everything from the common cold to cancer. Consider these facts:

- People who sleep seven or more hours a night have an infection rate of 18% when exposed to the common cold virus. Those who average five hours of sleep a night have a 50% infection rate.

---

71 Matthew Walker, *Why We Sleep: Unlocking the Power of Sleep and Dreams*, (Scribner; 1st edition, October 1, 2017), p. 162.

- People who sleep seven to nine hours a night the week before getting a flu shot generate a powerful antibody reaction, which equals a robust, healthy immune system. Those who slept less than seven hours a night produced 50% fewer antibodies. Immune cell counts are still affected *a full year later* after just a short dose of sleep restriction. Similar findings have been reported for hepatitis A and B vaccines.
- In cancer studies, sleep-deprived mice showed a 200% increase in both the speed and size of cancer cells. Tumors were visibly far more aggressive, spreading to surrounding tissue, organs, and bone, and death rates escalated in sleep-deprived animals.
- A single night of four hours of sleep eliminated 70% of the natural killer cells (powerful and necessary cells in our immune system, whose job it is to identify foreign elements, like cancer cells, and eliminate them) circulating in the immune system.
- A large European study tracking over 25,000 individuals showed that people sleeping six hours or less per night have a 40% increased risk of developing cancer. Lack of quality sleep is equal to a potent fertilizer for rapid growth of cancer cells. It's dangerous, and the link between sleep and cancer is so scientifically clear that the World Health Organization has officially classified nighttime shift work as a "probable carcinogen."[72]

Poor sleep wipes out otherwise healthy immune cells. Even one night of poor sleep robs us of much of our natural immune

---

72 All study stats taken from research reported in *Why We Sleep* by Matthew Walker, PhD.

resilience. Imagine what continual and constant poor sleep as a lifestyle does!

Sleep and Weight Gain

The science on the link between sleep and weight is irrefutable: If you don't get sufficient sleep, you will gain weight. There is brilliant research out there about the connection between sleep and appetite. In short, when we get less than adequate sleep, the hormone that signals we're full sharply decreases while the chemicals that produce that hungry feeling are amplified. It's like double jeopardy, creating a profound imbalance of hormonal food desire. Folks are far more ravenous on four or five hours of sleep a night than those who get a good night's sleep.

Short sleepers average an extra 300 calories per day, which might not sound like too big of a deal. But that equals an extra 70,000 calories per year, or an extra ten to fifteen pounds. Sound familiar? And it's not just that we eat more when we sleep less; we also make poorer food choices. Our cravings for all the bad (but oh-so-good) things—think ice cream, chocolate, chips, bread—increase by 30%–40% when our sleep is reduced by a few hours each night.

The epidemic of insufficient sleep is likely a key contributor to the epidemic of obesity. The less we sleep, the less energy we have and the more sedentary we become, all while having less willpower against the amplified bad food cravings we experience when tired. It's the perfect storm for weight gain, or as Walker calls it, the "perfect recipe for obesity."

But it's not all bad news! According to Walker:

> The encouraging news is that getting enough sleep will help you control body weight. We found that a full night of sleep repairs the communication pathway between deep-brain areas that unleash hedonic desires and higher-order brain regions whose job it is to rein in these cravings. Ample sleep can therefore restore a system of impulse control within your brain, putting the appropriate brakes on potentially excessive eating.[73]

So if you want to lose a few extra pounds—or a lot of extra pounds—make sure that a healthy sleep regimen is part of your weight-loss program.

Sleep and Your Gut Biome

We've already extensively discussed the importance of gut health, but did you know that the important flora in your gut microbiome only flourish when your body gets adequate sleep? When we don't get sufficient sleep, our body's nervous system circuits don't have a chance to calm and rebalance. This triggers the production of extra cortisol, a stress hormone you may have heard of before. That cortisol is a cultivator of bad bacteria in your gut, which prevents healthy food from absorbing and ultimately leads to gastrointestinal problems.

Put Down the Pills

> There does not seem to be one major organ within the body, or process within the brain, that isn't optimally

---

73 Matthew Walker, *Why We Sleep: Unlocking the Power of Sleep and Dreams*, (Scribner; 1st edition, October 1, 2017), p. 176.

enhanced by sleep (and detrimentally impaired when we don't get enough).[74]

Given the amazing, whole-body benefits of sleep, wouldn't it be something if our doctors started regularly prescribing sleep as part of our health regimen? Imagine leaving your doctor's office with a prescription in hand that requires you to prioritize getting eight hours of good sleep each night? Instead, millions of us leave with a prescription for sleeping pills, which is a whole different story.

There is currently no pill on the market, legal or not, that induces natural sleep. Any pill that helps you fall (or stay) asleep does not provide you with the same beneficial sleep that we've discussed in this chapter. The statistics about pills that induce sleep should make us think twice before taking them.

Here's just a glimpse into the dark side of sleeping pills: Ambien-induced sleep caused a 50% weakening of brain cell connections. This means that memory connections that are normally solidified during sleep are actually *erased*. Prescription sleep aids are strongly linked to significantly higher rates of infections and cancer. They're also linked to death; even occasional users (those who take eighteen or fewer pills per year) are 3.6 times more likely to die during the study window than non-users.[75] I urge you to do your own research and to be extremely careful before resorting to taking these dangerous drugs.

---

74 Matthew Walker, *Why We Sleep: Unlocking the Power of Sleep and Dreams*, (Scribner; 1st edition, October 1, 2017), p. 7.

75 Daniel F. Kripke, "The Dark Side of Sleeping Pills: Mortality and Cancer Risks, Which Pills to Avoid & Better Alternatives," March 2013, *http://www.darksideofsleepingpills.com.*

Struggling to Sleep? Try This

Sleep offers a remarkable arsenal of astonishing health benefits. But so many of us struggle to get a good night's rest! If you're trying to stay away from prescription sleep aids, what can you do to improve your sleep? There are many things outside of medication that can significantly improve sleep for many of us. Some of these may seem obvious and simple, yet they can make a meaningful difference. Here are some recommendations that can help you get your very best sleep:

1. **Try to stay on a consistent sleep schedule.** Whenever possible, go to bed and wake up at the same time every day. Contrary to popular wishful thinking, it is physically impossible to "make up for" missed sleep by "binging" on sleep during the weekend. If you tend to lose track of time, consider setting an alarm for bedtime each night. Make going to bed a priority. A consistent bedtime will train your body that it is supposed to get sleepy at that time each night and will greatly improve your ability to fall asleep.
2. **Avoid caffeine.** I know this is an unpopular suggestion, but caffeine is actually a powerful chemical stimulant that artificially mutes sleep signals in our brain. The consumption of caffeine has become such an unquestioned part of daily life that we do not realize the dangers of using (and abusing) this very-available psychoactive stimulant. The effects of this stimulant have a really long half-life, which means it can stay in your system for a full eight hours. Many people who think they have insomnia are simply unable to sleep due to the amounts of caffeine still in their systems.

3. **Create your ideal sleep atmosphere.** We get our best sleep when we're cool, dark, and comfy. Science says cooler is better, so turn that thermostat down at bedtime! We sleep best at temperatures between 65° and 67° Fahrenheit (18° and 19° Celsius). We also sleep best in the dark. Our brains are hardwired to sleep when it is dark and wake when there is even a bit of light. Our current industrialized schedules don't match that of the sun, however. If you struggle to sleep well, invest in some blackout curtains and keep your room really dark. An even more important sleep investment is a good mattress. We spend approximately a third of our lifetime in bed. If your mattress is more than seven years old or is not a comfortable fit for you, please research and buy a quality mattress! This is one of the most important investments you can make for your good health. Lastly, put down the device. That blue LED light that emits from your laptop, iPad, or phone inhibits your body's ability to produce its own melatonin. In fact, it suppresses natural melatonin production by more than double that of a regular yellow light bulb, delaying the onset of sleep by more than 90 minutes.
4. **Develop a relaxing bedtime ritual.** If you have children, you are probably very familiar with the importance of bedtime rituals. Think of all you do to create the proper environment to get a child to go to sleep. It's a whole event! This idea is equally important and works the same for adults. Spend time deliberately unwinding before you go to bed. Taking a hot bath actually helps cool your body's core temperature, enabling better sleep. Turn the lights down and listen to calming music. Read a book (but not on a device, see #3 above). Do some easy yoga stretches to work the tension out of

your body. Learn anxiety-reducing practices that help calm your mind and shelf the worries of the day, such as meditation. Whatever you do, do it nightly until it becomes a habit, signaling to both your body and your brain that it's time to prepare for sleep.

5. **See a specialist.** If your sleep problems persist, perhaps you have a diagnosable sleep disorder, such as sleep apnea or insomnia. If that's the case, you need professional help. Consider seeing a sleep medicine doctor, and not just your general provider, who has probably had surprisingly minimal sleep training.

Sleep really is the "Swiss army knife" in our optimal health toolkit. Figuring out my sleep issues was life-changing for me. Experiencing truly restorative sleep every night made an astonishing difference in how I felt, both physically and mentally. I also believe that it was the combination of improving my sleep, changing the foods I was eating, and getting off my medications that enabled me to improve my memory, which had been such a struggle after multiple surgeries the past few years. My wife says the change in my memory has been remarkable, and that my memory is now sharper than hers. This is a huge health victory for me.

They say that sleep strengthens our immune system, helps us regulate our appetites and impulses, contributes to cardiovascular health, improves brain function/memory, and even helps maintain a healthy microbiome in the gut. I'm a believer. Healthy sleep is the single most effective thing we can do for our overall health and wellness.

Now—go take a nap!

CHAPTER 3

REMOVE NSAIDS FROM YOUR DIET

David Meine

Aspirin, produced in 1897 by Felix Hoffman of the Bayer Company, was the first NSAID (nonsteroidal anti-inflammatory drug). Later, phenylbutazone and indomethacin were introduced. At that time, the mechanism of the action of these medications was unknown. Dr. John Vane eventually discovered that these medications work by inhibiting the production of prostaglandins, which promote inflammation and pain. After that discovery, the pharmaceutical industry was able to produce similar agents such as ibuprofen and naproxen, which we now know inhibit the enzyme cyclooxygenase (COX).

Here's a list of common NSAIDs:

- Advil / Motrin (ibuprofen)
- Aspirin
- Aleve (naproxen sodium)
- Celebrex

- Naprosyn (naproxen)
- Lodine (etodolac)
- Mobic
- Nalfon (fenoprofen)
- Daypro (oxaprozin)
- Ansaid (flurbiprofen)
- Cambia / Cataflam / Voltaren (diclofenac)
- COX-2 Inhibitors

The pharmaceutical industry actually recognizes all of these as "gateway drugs" because the damage they cause will eventually be the catalyst for many customers to move on to more potent prescription opioid painkillers. Since their inception, these companies knew NSAIDs caused severe damage to the mucosal barrier in the small intestine and colon, but the rest of us had no way of knowing. Gastroscopes couldn't reach that far, so doctors had no way to see the damage being caused until camera pills were invented. Once it was possible to swallow a camera, the damage being caused by NSAIDs was traceable and clear, but by that time, these medications had become ubiquitous. They'd become as much a part of our lives as chewing gum.

But NSAIDs are far more dangerous than gum! According to Dr. Gundry, who has done extensive research on the damage caused by NSAIDs and treated thousands of patients for this damage, "The more pain, the more you use NSAIDs—until you graduate to the big boys, the prescription painkillers. NSAIDs are both the number-one pharmaceutical seller and the number-one health menace. So, remember this: swallowing one Advil or Aleve is like swallowing a hand grenade. Also remember: the precursors of Advil and Aleve, ibuprofen and Naprosyn, were recognized as so dangerous when they were introduced in the

1970s that they were available only as prescription drugs."[76] I know this sounds dramatic, and Dr. Gundry's rhetoric is very strong. But all the research I've done on NSAIDs corroborates his memorable, if stark, description of them.

Although touted as an anti-inflammatory, NSAIDs actually increase inflammation, which you eventually feel as pain somewhere in your body. The more pain you feel, the more NSAIDs you take. It is truly a vicious cycle and one I lived for decades. The current state of my gut is proof.

Leaky gut syndrome

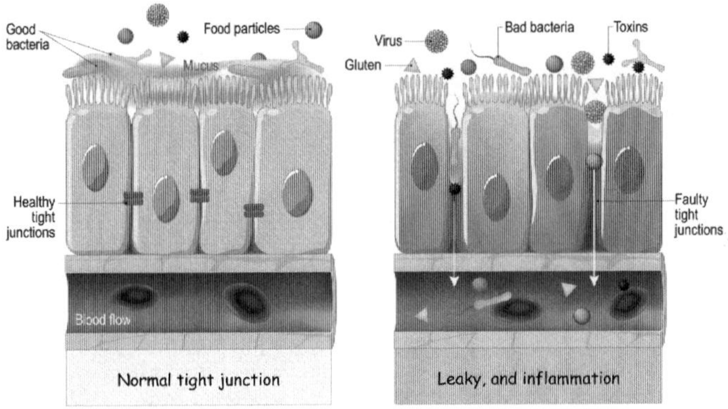

You've already read about my journey with NSAIDs in Chapter 9 of Part 1, and quite a bit about leaky gut syndrome in Chapter 10, but the above image is a great visual of what happens to our intestines when we ingest these medications. Once they loosen the tight junctions and pass into the bloodstream, they cause the immune system to attack our own cells, resulting in irritation, inflammation, and pain.

---

76 Dr. Steven Gundry, MD, *The Plant Paradox*, (Harper Wave; 1st edition, 2017), pp. 102-103.

All that Advil and Naproxen I took all those years never did treat the root cause of my pain. Instead, they made everything worse and created intense problems in my gut. One of those problems is my body's inability to tolerate many foods. Carla learned about an internationally-recognized doctor who offered extensive food sensitivity testing in her classes. Dr. Tom O'Bryan is a world expert on gluten, autoimmune diseases, and gut health. He helped us learn what gluten really does to our bodies. His clinic offers extensive testing, and I had a series of "Zoomers" blood analyses done in July 2020. The results confirmed Dr. Gundry's diagnosis of leaky gut and helped me better understand how ingesting NSAIDs or even a little bit of gluten was weakening those tight gap junctions and wreaking havoc on my body.

In the 192-page report, I was told that I have sensitivities to the following foods:

- Wheat
- Corn
- Egg yolk
- Egg white
- Dairy
- Soy
- Peanut
- Almond
- Macadamia
- Cashew
- Walnut
- Brazil nut
- Pistachio
- Pecan
- Salmon

- Trout
- Sardine
- Herring
- Pilchard
- Clam
- Quinoa
- Oats
- Rice
- Barley
- Rye
- Buckwheat
- Goat milk
- Sheep milk
- Camel milk
- Donkey milk

What in the world? Going through these results, my first thought was, *Is there anything even left to eat?* Granted, I don't drink a lot of donkey milk, but rice, wheat, corn, eggs, dairy, oats, and even salmon? I wouldn't wish this daunting list of food restrictions on anyone! Typing this list makes intense emotions of anger and frustration well up in me. I get angry tears from the realization that I have been suffering for sixty-four years due to a lack of knowledge and misinformation.

What does this revelation really mean? Why do I now have to deal with all of these food issues? Because I have been in a vicious cycle with a leaky gut. The leaky gut was causing inflammation in my body, so I took Advil or Naproxen to deal with the associated pain, which actually increased the inflammation, which increased the pain. And on and on. One of the results I get to live with now is a highly-restrictive food diet, as my gut simply can't tolerate many common foods.

Hopefully, by now, you're realizing what a true threat NSAIDs are to our health. However, you might also be thinking, *But I can't live without them!* Even if you don't take them nearly as often as I did over the years, how do you get through a bad headache day or the pain from tweaking your back at the gym this morning? Thankfully, there are some safe alternatives to popping ibuprofen every time you need help dealing with pain. Choosing one of these alternatives might achieve the same effects with much fewer unwanted reactions.

There are many other things you can do to relieve pain besides medicating. Let's consider things you can do to treat a headache. It's amazing how much is still unknown about headaches, but researchers are now suggesting that no matter the type of headache (stress headache, migraine, chronic headache, etc.), the treatment should be the same. Stress is a frequent contributor to the development of headaches. Relaxation techniques, like a long bath or meditation, can be helpful. There are some over-the-counter ointments and salves you can rub on your temples that many people say help reduce headache pain. There is even research that says acupuncture can be effective in reducing symptoms of chronic headache pain.

One of the most important things you can do to help eliminate any form of pain you are dealing with is to clean up your diet and eliminate NSAIDs. I didn't struggle with chronic headaches, but like many of you, I used to get the occasional headache. Since I have eliminated NSAIDs and cleaned up what I'm putting into my body, I haven't had a headache in well over two years. As for my other pain, which was devastating on a daily basis, it took between three and six months for the pain levels to drop dramatically. Be aware that it will take time for your body to begin to heal from the long-term damage that's been created, but it is worth the effort to live without chronic pain!

The medical industry is still in its infancy in regard to truly understanding leaky gut and its long-term effects (remember, it takes an average of seventeen years for the medical world to fully adopt new research). Right now, the experts don't all agree on leaky gut and how to treat it. This same industry also does not agree about NSAIDs and their detrimental effects. Carla and I are not medical doctors, and it is not our intention to diagnose, treat, cure, or recommend adjustments to any prescriptions or supplements that you use. You should always consult with your physician before embarking on any changes to your current treatment. But I strongly encourage you to consider eliminating NSAIDs.

I realize it seems like a big ask to stop taking NSAIDs. You might be reading this and thinking, as I did, that there is *no way* you can give up your Advil or Aleve. But I urge you to learn more about the devastating effects—including greatly increased pain in the long-term—of these drugs. Eliminating them from your diet won't be a quick fix. But it will be a long-term fix and one that is incredibly worth the effort.

WEIGHT LOSS IS JUST A PERK

Told by Carla Meine, with client's permission

I have a client who was referred to me by a friend who told her I could help her lose thirty-five pounds. I don't generally work with clients who are solely focused on weight loss, but Tammy (whose name has been changed at her request) had a strong WHY. She was tired of being miserable and was willing to commit to the big changes I was suggesting. I believed I could help her.

When I first meet with a client, I've already read the extensive intake form they've filled out, which means I have lots of additional questions for them. We usually spend ninety minutes together going over their life history, health challenges, current lifestyle, and what they're willing to do to change. While meeting with Tammy, I could tell she was highly motivated.

I also discovered that she was suffering from tinnitus (ringing in the ears) and joint pain, really struggled with sleeping, and had numbness in her toes. When you spend enough time with people, you can discover what is really going on! But Tammy was so focused on her weight loss woes that she had been a bit oblivious to the toll these other health issues were taking on her.

Tammy liked intermittent fasting, so it was easy to get her on a plan. She eats her first meal of the day between 11:00 a.m. and noon and finishes her last meal by 7:00 p.m. I gave her smoothie recipes to cover one of those meals, and it was really simple to work my other healthy recipes into the other meal. She would typically fix her large family roasted vegetables, some type of protein (chicken, fish, or beef), and a big salad. She'd just use a different dressing than they did. When the family wanted their pizza or pasta night, she'd just heat up some healthy leftovers for herself.

We started off by eliminating sugar, gluten, and dairy. Since she was highly motivated, she was able to be 100% compliant, and the weight just started coming off. After two months, she reported that she was sleeping better, something that always helps with weight loss. She was excited about the increased energy she was feeling. She also shared that her brain fog, which she hadn't initially told me about, was improving.

By the third month, the ringing in her ears was pretty much gone. She thought it must've been connected to the weight loss, but I explained that by removing foods that cause inflammation, it was lessening the inflammation in her brain, thus eliminating her tinnitus. She was thrilled.

When we met at four months, she had lost twenty pounds, the joint pain was gone (weight loss will always have a positive effect on joints), and she even noticed the numbness in her toes starting to get better. All was going well. She continued to lose weight and feel better every month.

It was at month six that this story really got good. Tammy called and shared that she had three bad days where she decided to eat a little sugar and gluten. The first night, it was some milk chocolate. Since we'd started working together, she had only had dark chocolate with at least 70% cocoa. But it was a night out with some friends, and the milk chocolate fondue just looked so good she couldn't resist having some.

That night, she noticed she struggled to get to sleep. She chalked it up to the caffeine in chocolate and didn't give it another thought. The next day, one of her kids had some candy on the kitchen counter. She thought, I'm doing so good. Surely a few pieces of this candy can't hurt! So she ate some. That night, it took her over an hour to get to sleep. Then she woke up in the middle of the night with her ears ringing, and she had a hard time getting back to sleep.

The next day, she was really tired. That night, the kids wanted pizza for dinner and brownies for dessert. Usually, she'd just make herself some leftovers and have one of the sugar- and gluten-free desserts on my website and be fine. This time, she decided that a couple of pieces of pizza and one small brownie surely wouldn't make that much of a difference. After all, she had hit her goal weight, and she deserved a reward.

But that reward came with a high price. Once again, she couldn't sleep. Her joints hurt. The numbness in her toes was even worse than it had been six months ago. When she woke again in the middle of the night with ringing in her ears, she was able to connect the dots. All of her symptoms were as bad as they had ever been, all from just three days of sugar and gluten.

Suddenly, it wasn't about weight loss anymore. She realized how great she had been feeling these past months and how much she missed it! Here she was, completely miserable again, even though she was thirty-five pounds lighter, just from three days of sugar and gluten.

The next day, she forced herself to wait until noon to drink her smoothie. Once she started eating sugar again, it became much more difficult to fast until noon. She made sure to eat some good veggies that day, a big salad, and a small portion of meat. That night, she fell right to sleep and didn't wake until the morning. That was all it took; she made the commitment to stay off sugar and gluten so that she could fully enjoy her life.

Tammy has stayed committed. We no longer talk regularly since she's met her goals, but we recently reconnected, and she told me she has even more energy and is sleeping even better now than she was when we were working together. She's kept the weight off, but that's just an added perk to the wonderful health benefits she continues to reap. For Tammy, choosing "eating to live" is worth it every single day.

LEVEL 3

CHAPTER 1

AN INTRODUCTION TO LEVEL 3

Carla Meine

Level 3 of *Eating to Live* is exciting as we progress from talking about all the things we won't do and start focusing on the things we *will* do on our journey to optimal health. This includes learning how to train our brains for long-term success and proper nutritional supplementation. Both are integral components of healthy living. Level 3 is also where we can try adding meats back into your meal planning.

Most of our clients love this phase of the program. They have missed their red meat and are excited to start adding it back into their diet. A word of caution, though—don't overdo it when adding meat. Keep it to four to ten ounces a day (depending on your size and gender), and keep track of how you feel when you add a particular meat. Your gut will process meats differently than someone else's. Maybe you find beef is just fine for you, but when you have pork, you have stomach issues. Or you did just fine with wild elk, but the beef caused constipation.

Tracking in your Eating to Live Journal is by far the most important part of your meal plan. Without tracking, you won't be able to figure out which foods help your system to function best. When you have a stomach issue, you can look back over the past one to three days and see what you ate. Look for patterns as to which foods are causing you discomfort.

When it comes to stomach issues, gas, bloating, and indigestion signal that something you've eaten (or overeaten) in the last few hours is causing the problem. If you have diarrhea or constipation, you need to look back at what you've eaten during the last two to three days and see if you can identify what is causing these issues. Once you find a potential culprit, simply remove that food from your meal plan for a few days and track how you feel. You truly are the only person that can discover the best foods for you to eat in order to achieve your optimal health.

In Level 3, we will add different types of meat to the food lists from Levels One and Two. Keep eating plenty of organic fruits and veggies! We can't stress enough how important organic fruits and vegetables are to your diet. One of our main goals is to remove as many toxins from your body as possible so that your liver can function at an optimal level (learn more about how important your liver is in the informative section below). If you keep introducing toxic pesticides in the foods you eat, your liver will continue to be overworked. This will manifest itself in a variety of health issues.

When you decide to move to Level 3, make sure the meat you add to your diet is beef that has been grass-fed and finished. This means the beef has been out in nature for its entire life, not just for short windows of time, eating what is natural and healthy for it to eat. Like Dr. Gundry says, not only is it true that you are what you eat, "You are what the thing you are eating ate." So be very picky about the meat you eat! We also like to add in organ meat, wild bison, venison, and elk. We will also add limited amounts of pork (humanely-raised), prosciutto, and lamb.

Level 3 foods include everything in Levels 1 and 2, plus meats. Here is the Level 3 Food Chart with the new food category listed.

Level 3

Vegetables	Peppers*	**Fruits**	**Seafood and Fish**	**Dairy Substitutes**
Arugula	Parsley	Apricots	Clams	Organic, full-fat coconut milk
Artichokes	Radicchio	Apples	Cod	Organic, un-sweetened nut milk
Asparagus	Radishes and leaves	Bananas	Crab	Almond milk
Avocado	Romaine lettuce	Blackberries	Halibut	Hazelnut milk
Acorn squash	Rutabaga	Blueberries	Herring	Hemp milk
Beets and beet greens	Scallions	Currants	Lobster	Yogurts made from coconut milk
Bok choy	Shallot	Cranberries	Mackerel	**Non-gluten Grains**
Beans, green	Squash	Cherries	Mussels	Almond four
Broccoli	Sweet potatoes	Dates	Oysters	Other nut flour
Brussel sprouts	Snow peas	Elderberries	Salmon	Amaranth

Bamboo shoots	Spinach	Figs	Sardines	Arrowroot
Chard	Seaweed	Grapes	Sea bass	Coconut flour
Chicory	Sea vegetable	Grapefruit	Shrimp	Cassava flour
Cilantro	Turnips and turnip greens	Goji berries	Trout	Flaxseeds/ flax
Collard greens	Tomatoes*	Honeydew melon	Tuna	Sorghum
Cabbage	Watercress	Kiwi	**Oils (cold-pressed)**	Tapioca
Celery	Water chestnuts	Lemon	Avocado oil	**Noodles**
Cucumber	Zucchini	Limes	Flax oil	Cappello's fettuccine
Carrots	Yams	Mango	Hemp oil	Pasta slim
Cauliflower	White potato (limit 1 per week)	Oranges	Olive oil (extra virgin)	Shirataki noodles
Chives	**Flavorings**	Pineapple	Nut oil	Kelp noodles
Dandelion greens	Coconut aminos	Pumpkin	MCT oil	Miracle noodles & Kanten pasta
Eggplant*	Herbs and spices	Pears	**Cooking Oils**	Miracle rice
Endive	Horseradish	Papaya	Avocado oil	Sweet potato noodles
Escarole	Himalayan sea salt	Peaches	Clarified butter/Ghee	Spaghetti squash noodles
Green peas (Green, split peas, black-eyed peas)	Mustard	Plums	Coconut oil	Zucchini and squash noodles
Garlic	Nutritional yeast	Pomegranates	Pecan oil	Rice
Hearts of palm	Pickles	Passion fruit	Sesame oil	**Bone Broth**

Kale	Sauerkraut	Prunes	**Sweeteners** (1 tsp. per day)	1 cup per day, gluten-free, organic
Lettuce (all but iceberg)	Sea salt (preferably iodized)	Raspberries	Honey	**Beverages**
Leeks	Tamari (gluten-free only)	Rhubarb	Just Like Sugar	Water
Mushrooms	Wasabi (gluten-free only)	Raisins	Real maple syrup	Club soda
Mustard greens		Strawberries	Molasses	Coffee (limit 2 cups per day)
Mizuna		Tangerines	Monk fruit	Tea (black, green, white, red root, oolong, match, herbal)
Onions		Watermelon	Sorghum	Yerba mate
Okra		Vinegars	Stevia	Kombucha tea
Olives		Any, if no added sugar	Swerve	**Chocolate**
			Xylitol	70% or greater, 1 oz. per day
Poultry**	Eggs** (pasture-raised only)	**Nuts & Seeds**** (if you can tolerate them)	**Meats***** (grass-fed, humanely-raised, or wild when possible)	

Chicken	Chicken	Tree Nuts • Almonds • Walnuts • Hazelnuts • Cashews • Brazil nuts • Pistachios • Macadamia nuts • Pecans • Chestnuts • Pinenuts	Beef	
Duck	Duck	Seeds • Sunflower • Pumpkin • Sesame • Flax • Chia • Psyllium	Bison	
Dove		Peanuts	Brain	
Goose		Tahini	Elk	
Pheasant		Sunflower butter	Gizzard	
Turkey		Almond butter	Heart	
			Kidney	
			Liver	
			Lamb	
			Pork	
			Sweet breads	
			Tongue	
			Veal	
			Venison	

**unless you have issues*

***Level 2 food group additions*

****Level 3 food group additions*

Your Detox Super-Organ: The Liver

Sugar, gluten, and all the other unhealthy foods we tend to love (fried foods, processed foods, alcohol, etc.) are really bad for you, but where they really wreak havoc is in the liver. This "super-organ" literally performs hundreds of jobs all day. Andrea Nakayama explains its function very well:

> The liver is the primary filter or gatekeeper in our bodies, and this is why some say it's the number-one reason for illness. The functions can be broken down into three main categories (blood filtering, detoxification, and bile synthesis and secretion), but the liver actually has hundreds of functions, some of which include the following: The liver is responsible for the regulation of fat storage; it certainly cleanses the blood; it discharges waste; it neutralizes and destroys poisons; it manufactures new body proteins; it metabolizes alcohol; it manages the chemicals in the blood; it aids in digestion through the production of that bile; it produces immune factors; it helps to remove bacteria from the blood; it stores vitamins, minerals, and sugars; it maintains hormone balance; it controls the production and secretion of cholesterol, and it's responsible for regenerating its own damaged tissue.[77]

Wow, that really is one busy and amazing organ! A healthy liver is integral to maintaining a healthy gut. It's the largest internal organ in our bodies, and it's the most important organ when it comes to detoxification. Proper nutrition and regulating our diet is how we do cleanup from the outside in. Maintaining

---

77 Andrea Nakayama, Liver Intensive, April 2020.

a healthy liver is how we instigate cleanup from the inside out. The challenge for the liver is what we put into our bodies. The food we eat, the beverages we drink, and the toxins we breathe in all have to go through the liver. When we overtax the liver by consuming bad foods (especially processed foods), all our systems are affected. Our gut microbiome is especially jeopardized when the liver is unable to filter properly, which can lead to leaky gut. And we know that this can lead to many miserable health issues down the road.

Your Eating to Live Meal Plan Facilitates Liver Health

By this point in your *Eating to Live* journey, you've eliminated most foods that typically tax the liver, such as sugars, processed foods, and unhealthy fats. Too much sugar stresses the liver. Simple carbohydrates make the liver work overtime. Our bodies convert excess sugars into fat, which is stored in the liver. This is the major indicator of heart disease and why sugar is actually a bigger factor in heart disease than fats. But fats are also harmful to the liver. If you've ever heard of a liver cleanse, they remove many fats from the diet to give the liver a break. When the liver isn't processing and storing extra fats, it can actually focus on its other jobs, like detoxing your body (remember, there is a big difference between healthy fats, like avocado, and unhealthy fats, like french fries).

There are other important things to avoid that put undue stress on the liver. Overeating makes the liver work triple time. Consuming too much enzyme-deficient food taxes the liver. NSAIDs cause toxic buildup in the liver that inhibits its ability to function. Alcohol inflames the liver, and it's much more difficult for the liver to properly filter when it is inflamed. When inflammation is combined with being clogged up with fat, which leads to cirrhosis or the hardening of the liver cells, then the liver can no longer regenerate itself. Lack of exercise means the liver has to be in charge of toxin elimination that should be happening through the lungs and skin. Yep, sweating when you work out plays an important role in getting rid of body toxicity!

Your liver is the primary site for poison (toxin) control in your body. Every single thing you eat and every toxin that enters your body—whether through your digestive tract, your respiratory tract, or your skin—passes through your liver before entering the bloodstream for general circulation. Your liver is working on ridding your body of harmful substances around the clock. The health of the whole body is reflected in how well your liver is able to perform its role of detoxification.

Staying committed to a healthy and nutritious diet is crucial for liver health, and because the liver affects every other system in your body—especially your gut—you'll want to stay committed to your new nutritious lifestyle. A healthy liver plus a healthy gut microbiome equals a healthier, happier you.

CHAPTER 2

TRAIN YOUR BRAIN FOR OPTIMAL HEALTH

David Meine

"Thoughts are energy. And you can make your world or break your world by thinking."

—SUSAN L. TAYLOR

Do you have a hobby or pastime you are passionate about? Something you spend hours and hours doing, simply because you love it? Take a moment and think about how much time you spent learning and studying this hobby or skill.

In the space below, please answer the questions about your hobby:

- How many hours have you invested in this hobby (your best guess)? ______________
- How much money have you spent on this hobby/ developing this skill (taking classes, buying equipment, etc.)? ______________

If this hobby or skill is something you have done for many years and spent hundreds of hours doing, you have developed a pretty robust, subconscious, automatic memory for it. Or, in other words, much of it probably comes very naturally to you now. Unlike when you were first learning to participate in your hobby, it likely requires much less mental focus.

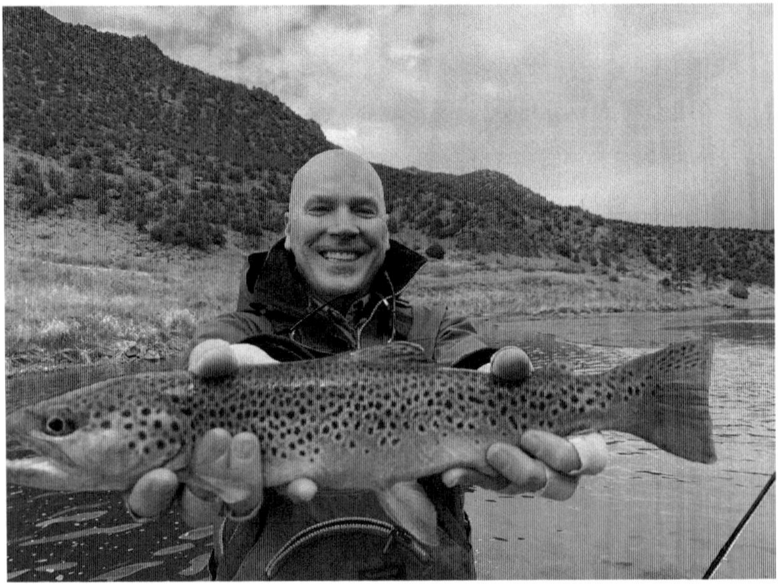

Let me give you a personal example: I have spent hundreds of hours developing a motion with my right hand, arm, and shoulder that whips the line with a fly attached while casting a fly-fishing rod. I whip it backward at a one o'clock position and forwards at a nine o'clock position. This casting is modified based on the wind, width of the stream or river, and the thickness of the foliage nearby. I have done this for so many years that I now barely even think about those things while fishing. As I hunt for where the fish are most likely feeding, my body motions are automatically dictated by the brain training I have done in the past during all those hours of practice.

Recently, I took up a modified form of fly fishing called Euro nymphing. Casting a Euro nymphing fly rod is totally different from traditional fly fishing. All of the brain training that is stored in my subconscious brain from regular fly fishing created huge issues. All that automatic memory was really messing me up! I finally hired a guide to see why the casting was so difficult. Once he walked me through, step by step, how to cast this new style, it took six hours of constant casting, being coached by the guide at my side, until my subconscious brain would cooperate. Over time, this new technique will become second nature. But it takes frequent, consistent practice and a highly engaged brain for this process to become automatic.

It would have been much easier to continue to use the traditional form I was already comfortable with. But I chose to put in the effort required to do this because of *why* I fish. Can you see the pure joy on my face in the picture of me holding the fish? Besides being with my family, this is truly my happy place. I keep some of the fish I catch, and Carla turns them into a healthy and tasty meal. Most of the time, however, I practice catch-and-release. Every precaution is taken to not harm the fish. The thrill comes with reeling in the fish and not losing it before it's been netted. I chose to learn Euro nymphing because this new technique would allow me to catch more fish, thus enjoying the thrill of catch-and-release more often.

After consistent practice, which retrained my brain, I now catch three times the number of fish using this Euro nymphing style. It took some work and came with a whole slew of unexpected challenges.

Whenever we work to learn something new, or undo a bad habit, or train or retrain our brain in any way, it's going to come with challenges. That brings me to the most important question of all: *Is it worth it?* The answer to that question depends on the strength of your WHY. I'm sure it's obvious that, for me, fly fishing, in general, is definitely worth it! Spending many hours learning and incorporating a new style of casting was worth it three times over because I catch three times more fish in the same stretch of river!

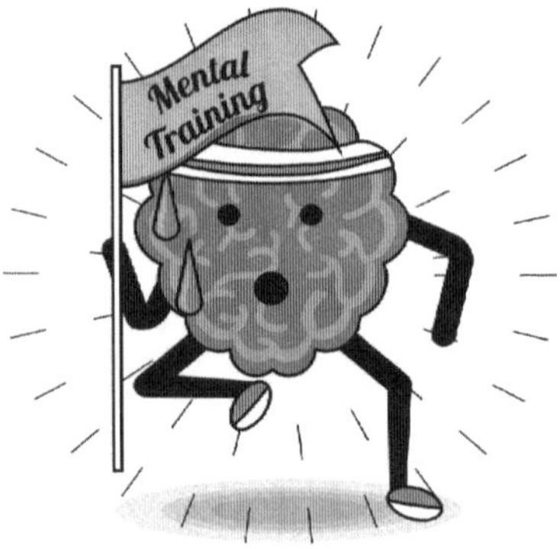

Although our focus here is on achieving optimal health, brain-training skills are applicable to many other areas of life as well. This chapter has powerful tools that can truly transform your health and create a quality life that can inspire those around you. Any time you want to modify your brain, you can employ some "mental training" and really make a difference.

Mental Training

How many thoughts would you guess that you think each day? Scientists have just recently found a way to identify and count separate thoughts, discovering that the average person has 6,200 separate thoughts each day.[78] These thoughts affect the many daily choices we make. They also affect our behaviors

78 Jason Murdock, "Humans Have More than 6,000 Thoughts per Day, Psychologists Discover," Newsweek, 15 July 2020, *https://www.newsweek.com/humans-6000-thoughts-every-day-1517963.*

and habits, especially since the great majority of our thoughts happen at a subconscious (psychologists sometimes refer to this as unconscious) level. This means your brain has a powerful influence on appearance, mood, weight, stress levels, and overall health.

So, how do we create a brain-friendly environment that will allow us to edit unhealthy food and beverage habits? Let me share two brain-training experiences that I had recently. I grew up on Coca-Cola products. I started young and didn't stop—I drank several delicious, ice-cold Cokes every day, and my addiction level was strong! Then, seven years ago, I wrote an article about sugar. It was no longer possible to avoid the reality of what I was ingesting, and it motivated me to overcome my habit of drinking Coke. I utilized a self-hypnosis process that I had learned and stopped drinking Coke over a sixty-day period.

A couple of years ago, however, I started drinking Coke Zero. I rationalized that I could enjoy the flavor of my old friend Coke without all the bad sugars. Of course, there were two big issues I was trying hard not to think about, as Coke Zero is far from healthy. Aspartame and caffeine are super bad villains in the fight for good health and great sleep. Plus, Coke Zero is highly addictive, just like its cousin, Coke.

As I was researching brain training while writing this book, my Coke Zero habit came to mind. I've eliminated so many of my negative health behaviors, but I really wanted to hold onto this one. Couldn't I keep this one small thing? Just thinking about the satisfying sizzle of bubbles when I open the can and the sound of that delicious brown liquid as I pour it over my favorite pebble ice makes me happy (that's red-flag, addiction-level happiness, by the way!).

But I knew that the reality was that this daily habit was affecting my health. I began researching to see if there were any articles, studies, or protocols for regular people like me who were simply trying to kick a habit. There were none to be found. I decided to develop a simple brain-training protocol that anyone could use when trying to train the brain.

First, I needed to do what I call a "brain edit" and find a positive behavior to replace the negative behavior. I decided to substitute my Coke Zero beverage with water. I'm sure you are thinking what I was thinking: "Water is *boring*." I am not nearly as excited to drink water as I was to have my lovely Coke Zero. So, I try to find ways to make my water more exciting, like cutting up fresh limes and squeezing them into my water. I also frequently acknowledge mentally and out loud that the behavior change is to completely stop drinking Coke Zero and replace it with water. My brain needs to hear it and think it in order to realize I really am truly committed to changing this habit and breaking homeostasis.

Replacing a behavior as comfortable and addictive as this one definitely takes a strong WHY, so I employed the Why-How-What Worksheet and determined the WHY, HOW, and WHAT of breaking this particular habit.

1. **Behavior to Modify or Change:** Stop drinking Coke Zero.
2. **WHY:** Coke Zero's caffeine has dramatically affected the quality of my sleep, and the aspartame has negative effects on my health.

3. **HOW:** When offered a choice of beverages, I will select water (I will always ask for lemon slices if available).
4. **WHAT:** I will do the daily visualization script that helps edit out the bad behavior.
   WHAT: I will not buy Coke Zero at grocery stores or convenience stores.
   WHAT: I will not let others that are drinking Coke Zero affect my commitment.

Having a plan is an important step in changing my behavior and training my brain. The most important part of brain training, however, is daily accountability. How would I make sure I truly employed these behaviors every day? I chose to use my iPhone Notes App to record each day's compliance. I remember so vividly the end of the first successful day with no Coke Zero. I enthused to Carla, "I went this whole day without a Coke Zero! Hurray!" She laughed and gave me that look, like, "Wow, that's a pretty big deal about a whole day without your soda!"

But I knew it truly WAS a big deal! I typed "Day 1: DRY!" into my app. At the time, we were on vacation and eating dinner out each night. Each dinner became a test to see if I could replace the Coke Zero with water and lemons. Each time the server asked for our beverage order, I would respond with, "Water, please. And do you have lemon slices?"

Each night, I would record in my app and tell Carla that I was, "Dry another day!" She would laugh and say, "Great job." By the end of the week, she realized that I was serious about this change. I realized I was serious, too. The visualization exercise was working, and my verbal affirmations were imprinting new neural pathways that were literally changing my thoughts. The

Why-How-What was clearly defined, and it was working. I was being accountable and recording my progress every day.

Guess what? I have been "dry" ever since! I am sleeping better. Unfortunately, I can't measure how eliminating aspartame from my diet has improved my health. But I absolutely believe that eliminating Coke Zero, with all its chemicals and unnatural ingredients, is improving my overall health and wellness. It's amazing what you can achieve once the brain believes. Almost everything becomes possible.

My second example is about utilizing brain training when learning something new. I have always wanted to learn to play the piano. I have dreams of playing for my family and envision them gathering around the piano on holidays and singing along as I accompany them. I requested a digital piano for Christmas last year and began taking lessons. Learning to play has been a tremendous challenge for me. This is essentially the opposite of what I was describing at the beginning of this chapter with fly fishing, which I've spent thousands of hours practicing. When it comes to playing the piano, I have zero subconscious automatic memory to draw from. It is hard! At a recent piano lesson with my teacher, Janelle, I was reminded about this brain-training technique.

Janelle was teaching me about musical phrasing. In essence, songs are composed of individual sentences or phrases. She told me I should start in the middle of the piece of music and work on one of these phrases. She said I had to be able to play that particular sentence, or phrase, five times in a row without making a mistake. Once I was able to do that, I could move on. "Why is that necessary?" I asked her, wanting to just start at the beginning and work my way through.

"You need to rewire your brain memory and train your brain how to do it correctly," she answered. Janelle picked a spot in the music that I was having particular difficulty with. "Work on just this part here until you can do it error-free five times in a row."

I followed her suggestion and found that my playing improved dramatically. I committed to practicing in this manner. Learning to play the piano is out of my comfort zone and requires a lot of mental effort, but I have a very strong WHY statement—to be able to play for my family and friends—that keeps me motivated to practice consistently. I can almost feel the connections happening in my brain when I practice in this way. And it shows in my playing, too.

Your Brain Is the Gatekeeper of Your Comfort Zone

First, we need to acknowledge why the brain will sabotage our efforts to improve our health when we try to change negative habits or implement new behaviors. Isn't our brain on our side?

In Chapter 2 of Level 1, I spoke about the brain being in homeostasis. Most of the 6,200 thoughts we have each day are part of our subconscious brain, whose job it is to reinforce and regulate our life. Think about how much of your life is "on autopilot"—breathing, body temperature, heartbeat, etc. Imagine if we had to consciously think about every one of our systems and regulate them. It would be overwhelming!

The subconscious mind has a homeostatic impulse. It works to keep your body temperature stable and balance the hundreds of chemicals in your billions of cells so that it all works in harmony. When we do something that interrupts homeostasis, or the status quo, the brain balks. It causes you to feel emotionally and physically uncomfortable whenever you try to do something new or different and change established patterns of behavior. That's its job.

This is why training the brain is so critical! All of our habits and patterns are stored in the subconscious mind. It knows your comfort zones and works to keep you in them. However, the subconscious mind obeys what the conscious mind tells it to. Through brain editing, accountability practices, and journaling practices such as the Why-How-What Worksheet, we have the power to literally rewrite the script and *change our brains*. Yes, replacing a negative behavior with a positive behavior is very difficult to do. But *it is absolutely doable!*

B-R-A-I-N

Let's go through a helpful acronym for BRAIN:

B is for BELIEVE. The first step in editing the brain is to believe. Believe that you can make the necessary change to create a new, healthy, and lasting habit.

Have you ever known someone who defied the odds? Perhaps someone who was given a horrible diagnosis and slim chance of survival, someone who should have died, given their circumstances, yet they overcame? Belief plays an important role here. If you believe you can overcome, you'll be much more inclined to do the things you don't want to do but are necessary and beneficial for your health.

In my own cancer battles, the belief that I could do it, that I could beat it, was so integral. This belief is powerful. It helps us to fight, to cope, to overcome, and to find meaning in the battle. As one doctor put it, "I… deal with cancer patients on a daily basis. I see patients that have a positive attitude about their cancer, and they either are cured or expand their life considerably compared to others that gave up the first day after they find out the news."[79] What we believe influences our behavior, and our behavior influences our quality of life.

"What you believe, you can achieve" is perhaps an over-used idiom, the sort of inspirational quote painted on the hall in the local junior high. But it's truer than many of us jaded adults think. What do you truly believe you are capable of? I believe you have the power to live the life you truly want. The brain is so powerful, and all we have to do is start with changing our beliefs.

79 Taz, "Positive Healing Through My Mind," The Secret TV, *https://www.thesecret.tv/stories/positive-healing-mind/.*

"Strength is the matter of a made up mind."
—JOHN BEECHER

"He who believes is strong; he who doubts is weak. Strong convictions precede great actions."
—J. F. CLARKE

"I was always looking outside myself for strength and confidence but it comes from within."
—ANONYMOUS

"Believe that life is worth living and your belief will help create the fact."
—WILLIAM JAMES

"Man is what he believes."
—ANTON CHEKHOV

"You can do a thing only if you have the belief that it can be done."
—ANONYMOUS

"It's what you choose to believe that makes you the person that you are."
—KAREN MARIE MONING

R is for RESIST. The greatest burden that we carry in our brain is self-sabotage. Negative thought patterns begin when we are children and seem to grow with us as we age. What does it take to resist sabotage from ourselves and others?

Get off the couch. Exercise is the fastest way to release endorphins that will help you resist negative thoughts. Nothing clears and calms the head faster than exercising. Every time I spend thirty minutes or more focused on some form of exercise, I know for a fact that I am improving the quality of my life and helping my brain to perform its best. Spending time exercising is something you won't regret, even if you don't feel like you have thirty minutes to spare. Get off the couch and get those happy endorphins flowing!

Just say no. When you're trying hard to make healthy choices, it can be so easy to get derailed by well-intentioned people. I can't even count how many times I've visited friends or family and have been confronted with sugar in its many forms. "Come on, just have one piece, David!" or, "I made them fresh today, surely one cookie can't hurt?" Somehow, it makes people happy if you eat their food, so it takes some serious resolve. I've learned to begin with a smile and a polite but very firm, "No, thanks." I then try to change the subject and the situation with a question about one of their interests outside of baking delicious cookies. If I can get them talking about themselves, they forget that I politely rebuffed their delicious offer.

Although most people truly are well-intentioned, there are sometimes those who feel threatened by your noticeably improving health. They might even try to intentionally sabotage your efforts. This topic could be a whole book of its own, but just be aware that this might happen and resolve to resist! Each time you flex your resistance muscles, they get stronger. Resistance is key to training your brain in new habits and patterns.

A is for ACCOUNTABILITY. Throughout this book, I have referred to the importance of creating ways that you can be accountable for your goals and brain-training efforts. There are many ways to do this. Journaling is a powerful and important way to hold yourself accountable. Doing something highly visible—like marking each day you successfully go without eating sugar with a bright-red lipstick checkmark on your mirror—is also effective. Or, you can simply use the notes app on your phone and mark each successful day with a little "Yay, me!" celebration as I did with my Coke Zero habit.

If possible, find someone else that helps hold you accountable. Research by the American Society of Training and Development (ASTD) found that there is a 65% greater chance of meeting an objective if you have committed to someone in addition to yourself that you are going to do so. Even better, if you set up specific "accountability appointments" with the person to whom you've committed, your chances of success in reaching your objective increase by 95%![80]

A study about exercise conducted by Stanford University found that simply by receiving a check-in phone call once every two weeks asking about goal progress increased the amount of exercise participants did by an average of 78%. And, those same study participants were still exercising at the increased level eighteen months after the study (and the check-in calls)

80 Thomas Oppong, "This Is How to Increase the Odds of Reaching Your Goals by 95%," Pocket, 1 January 2017, *https://getpocket.com/explore/item/this-is-how-to-increase-the-odds-of-reaching-your-goals-by-95.*

had ended.[81] They'd trained their brains and formed a new habit.

As author Dennis Waitley said, "There are two primary responses in life: to accept conditions as they exist or accept the responsibility for changing them."[82] Ultimately, we have the power to make lasting and meaningful changes in our lives. We take accountability once we accept the fact that we can edit a negative behavior and replace it with a life-changing, positive behavior.

I is for INGENUITY. The brain is so amazing in what it can inspire us to accomplish. According to the dictionary, the definition of "ingenuity" is the quality of being clever, original, and inventive. It means you are innovative and creative. In the eighties, there was a TV show called *MacGyver*, and the main character was known for his amazing ingenuity. He could thwart the enemy with little more than a paperclip and some duct tape. I eagerly watched each episode to see what innovative yet simple solution he would come up with next.

Throughout my life, I have been called a MacGyver. I can typically figure out how to solve many of the problems that I face. This has been helpful in my business and my personal life, but it's never been more important than it has been during my journey toward optimal health. If I had simply taken

---

81 Melissa McAllister, "The Power of Accountability Weight Loss," Melissa Made Online, *https://melissamadeonline.com/2017/05/26/the-power-of-accountability-in-weight-loss/.*

82 Dennis Waitley, as quoted on Hungry Faces, 4 June 2020, *https://hungryfaces.me/2020/06/04/there-are-two-primary-choices-in-life-to-accept-conditions-as-they-exist-or-accept-the-responsibility-for-changing-them-denis-waitley.*

everything at face value that all the doctors have said to me over the past two decades, I would not have the life I have today. I might not even be alive today. I had to be proactive as my own best advocate and use all the ingenuity I could muster as I researched alternatives to harmful prescriptions full of side effects that only masked the symptoms. It takes hard work and commitment and a great investment (another wonderful "I" word) of time and effort. But the payoff has been immense.

You might be thinking, "Well, I'm no MacGyver! How does ingenuity apply to me?" It's easy to sit back and watch others' ingenuity and to complement their ability to creatively problem-solve while denying your own ability to do so. Everyone's brain sees the world and solves problems differently, but I maintain that you are 100% capable of using creativity and out-of-the-box thinking to solve your problems. I urge you to challenge the status quo. Ask questions. Do your research. Dig deep and find alternative solutions. No one will advocate for your health the way that you can.

Ingenuity is key to successful brain training. Only you can come up with solutions and systems that best work for you as you work toward daily healthy habits. Accountability requires ingenuity.

N is for NEXT. Don't stop now! Instead, think of the next brain edit you'd like to accomplish. Stacking successful brain edits on top of each other can create truly sustainable possibilities for greatness throughout our lives. Poor habits, especially those that affect the health of our bodies and brains, keep us from truly enjoying life to its fullest. Each time we can replace a bad habit with a healthy habit, we get closer to achieving our optimal health.

Let's take a moment and actually do a simple brain-training exercise. Please use these pages as a workbook and write your answers to the following questions:

1. What is your next step? Hopefully, you have completed your WHY statement from the earlier chapter and have picked your first brain edit behavior that will turn a negative into a positive. If not, take a moment now and do so here. If you've already completed your WHY, please review it and use this page as a chance to update or modify it specifically to your goal of achieving optimal health.

   WHY I want to create my optimal health: ______________

   ____

   ____

   HOW I am going to create my optimal health: _________

   ____

   ____

   WHAT I am specifically going to do to create my optimal health: ______________________________________

   ____

   WHAT I am specifically going to do to create my optimal health: ______________________________________

   ____

   WHAT I am specifically going to do to create my optimal health: ______________________________________

   ____

2. Next, write down a brain edit goal that will start you on the path to optimal health. (Keep it simple—something

like drinking water at meals, sleeping eight hours a night or abstaining from sugary snacks, for example.): _____

____

3. Next, I want you to experience a visualization exercise. A visualization exercise is a powerful way to train your brain and override homeostasis. The best way to do visualization exercises is through mindful meditation. It just takes a few minutes, and this is a healthy, positive way to rescript your brain messaging. You can easily record this script yourself on the Voice Memo App on your smartphone, or you can listen to this script recorded in my voice on the *Eating to Live* website.[83]
   Take a deep breath and hold for the count of three, then exhale. Do this three times so you can relax your body and mind. Then, start listening to a recording of the script on the following page (yours or mine) to do this visualization exercise.

83 You can access this visualization at eatingtolive.com/book/. There are also a number of other visualization scripts available for you to access through your ETL membership.

Creating Optimal Health Visualization Script

Every day in every way, you have a powerful desire to be fit, healthy, and active.

Writing down your goal will begin the process of creating a positive belief cycle.

The next twenty-eight days of visualizing *(your goal)* will give you the mental strength that will help you create your optimal health.

You will become more aware of the many positive reasons to create your optimal health.

Any past barriers that have held you back from creating your optimal health are now dissolving and disappearing.

Every day that you do this visualization exercise, you will become more and more relaxed as you strengthen your belief to achieve your optimal health.

Your attitude grows more positive each passing day. Each day you will feel healthier. You are focused on *(your goal).*

You do this because you want to be healthier.

You do this because you want to feel stronger and live life more fully. You have a powerful desire to be healthy.

As you stay focused on *(your goal),* you will begin to notice changes in health.

Each day, you begin to feel the way you want to feel—strong, energetic, and vigorous.

You are now creating new ways of thinking about yourself and your health.

You are emerging with a wonderful awareness of your enjoyment of living.

Your body's natural process for creating healthy energy and vitality keeps you feeling great.

Your body thrives on your new positive mental attitude.

You find so much pleasure in being good to yourself.

You now focus on taking the best possible care of your body, both inside and out.

As each day passes, your inner mind becomes convinced that you truly want to create your optimal health.

This new belief about creating your optimal health is making a vivid, deep, and permanent impression on your subconscious mind.

And each day in your daily life, you become more and more aware of a wonderful feeling of personal confidence.

You gain confidence in the realization that each day brings you one step closer to achieving (your goal).

For each day is a vital step in problem-solving and changing your behavior.

By creating your optimal health, you will enjoy a fuller, richer, and more expressive life.

Each day you will become more confident, strong, consistent, rock-solid, and dedicated to creating your optimal health.

As your belief grows that you can improve your health, you will realize how powerful your mind can be in creating those positive changes that you desire.

Every day, the conscious and subconscious minds are in constant conflict. Most of us know basic truths about health and fitness. But knowing and doing are different things! It is so much easier to watch TV for four hours a day[84] (believe it or not, that is the actual amount of television that the average adult in the US watches daily) than to spend time and effort consciously working to improve our health.

But, a tiny spark can change all of that. It could be as simple as, "I will not drink one more unhealthy beverage." The spark is a belief that you can *choose* not to drink that beverage. Then, make a plan, and record every day that you're successful. Then, do the same thing the next day, and then the next day. The subconscious mind will begin to resist the edit and needs to see consistency. Accountability equals a much greater rate of consistency. Once you do this long enough, your brain seems to catch on, and it will stick. That belief becomes habitual behavior, and that behavior can become years of healthy, high-quality life.

---

84 "Television and Health," California State University, https://www.csun.edu/science/health/docs/tv&health.html.

CHAPTER 3

SUPPLEMENT YOUR FOOD WITH PROPER NUTRITION

Carla Meine

Do you currently take any supplements? Or do you believe, like so many people do, that supplements just make for expensive urine? I used to have that opinion, thinking that my body didn't really absorb much, that I was flushing most of the benefits away. Before he started measuring their effects, Dr. Gundry believed that as well. But after working with him for over three years and watching our own blood work change for the better, I'm convinced that the foods we eat don't have enough nutritional value to really heal the body without proper supplementation.

A supplement is just as its name describes; it is meant to be supplementary to a nutritious diet. No matter how many supplements you take, it doesn't replace the value of a healthy and nutritious salad of leafy greens. But the sad truth is that it is fairly impossible to get all the nutrients we need from food alone. Our fruits, vegetables, and grains are being grown in soil that has been depleted of the vitamins and minerals we need.

This fact was published in a US Senate document clear back in 1936,[85] which was before anyone had begun to think of genetically modifying food or the use of chemical fertilizers, pesticides, and biocides, which have sadly become the accepted norm in America. It was confirmed clear back in 2003 that our soil was significantly more depleted than it was in 1940.[86] This means that if you live in the US, even the healthiest eater simply isn't getting all of the minerals and nutrients they need from food alone.

In Level 3, we begin to add supplements to your healthy diet in order to reduce any bodily inflammation and repair the leaky gut that plagues so many of my clients.

Dietary supplements—and recommendations about supplements—can be found everywhere. Sifting through the options and the information can be overwhelming. Supplements also come in many forms, including pills, powder, or liquid. But regardless of form, the goal is to supplement your diet so that you get the right nutrients.

So, what supplements do you need to add to your meal plan? That's a tough question, and the answer is different based on each individual's situation. Your body's supplementation needs

---

85 United States Government, "Senate document #264, 74th Congress, 2nd Sessions, 5 June 1936," 26 March 2021, *https://www.prismnet.com/~lenb/centurynutrition/senate264.htm.*

86 D. Thomas, "A study on the mineral depletion of the foods available to us as a nation over the period 1940 to 1991," *Nutrition and Health* 17(2):85-115, 2003.

will be different from mine. Journaling remains incredibly important as you start adding supplements. This is ultimately how you will determine which supplements and what amounts work for you. You'll want to add one at a time, wait several days, and pay attention to your body, especially your bowel movements, to make sure the supplement you've added is good for you. As with all of my recommendations, you should work with your doctor to figure out what supplements are lacking in your body.

Because everyone is so different, it's impossible to list exactly what you need, but I can share which supplements almost everyone is deficient in. The following are the vitamins and supplements that pretty much everyone needs and feels noticeable benefits from when they add them to their daily regimen.

Vitamin D3 (the Sunshine Vitamin)

The most common supplement that is deficient in most of my clients is vitamin D. This was also the first supplement that Dr. Gundry increased for both David and me. This vitamin is necessary for our bodies to be able to absorb calcium and phosphorus, which keep our bones strong. But equally important is the boost it gives our immune systems. It also strongly benefits mood and heart health. We need more vitamin D than we think. According to Gundry, most Americans have very low levels of vitamin D. He estimates that of his patients from California, where there is plenty of sunshine, 80% are vitamin D deficient. If a patient has an autoimmune issue, that percentage increases to 100%.[87] We simply don't get enough D vitamins through foods and exposure to sunshine alone.

Vitamin D is an easy one to add that rarely has any bad side effects. Start by adding 5,000 IUs of vitamin D3 a day and then see what happens (D3 increases vitamin D levels overall in the blood more effectively than other D vitamins, which makes it the recommended form). For my clients that have been diagnosed with an autoimmune disease, I recommend starting with 10,000 IUs a day. When you get your bloodwork done at your next appointment, ask your doctor to check your vitamin D levels. I like to get my clients above 70 ng/ml, but work with your doctor to see what they recommend.

The B Vitamins

Most of my clients are dealing with leaky gut syndrome. This means the microbiome in their gut has been compromised. Because many B vitamins are produced by good gut bacteria, these clients are usually deficient in their B vitamins. Vitamin B complex is composed of eight B vitamins, and they are the building blocks of a healthy body, directly impacting energy levels, brain function, and cell metabolism. Taking B vitamins can also lower elevated cholesterol levels. Vitamin B is water-soluble, which means they do not stay in the body for long and cannot be stored. This makes daily supplementation of B vitamins essential.

---

87 Dr. Steven Gundry, MD, *The Plant Paradox*, (Harper Wave; 1st edition, 2017), p. 275.

I recommend taking a 1,000-microgram methylfolate tablet each day and putting 1,000 micrograms of methyl B12 under your tongue daily. Since this is a fairly safe supplement to add, the only caution is that if you notice increased depression or excitability, you should stop taking them.

Omega-3s

Another important supplement that provides a whole host of benefits are omega-3 fatty acids. These are also great for leaky gut, as they help repair your gut wall. Studies show that most people are profoundly deficient in omega-3s. This is especially worrisome because omega-3s are directly related to brain health. The brain is approximately 60% fat, so it makes sense that increasing your fatty acids would have a positive effect on your brain. Studies show that the higher the levels of omega-3 fats in your blood, the bigger your brain is and the better your memory is.[88]

I encourage my clients to take 1,000 mgs of DHA a day. To get that much DHA from a typical 1,400-mg fish oil capsule with 980 mgs of omega-3, you need to take four soft gels daily. It may seem like a lot, but I've seen remarkable results when my clients increase their intake of omega-3s. So many clients are experiencing brain fog and memory issues when we first start working together. Watching that brain fog lift and their memory improve as we remove sugars and gluten and add healthy supplements like fish oil is very rewarding!

Vitamin C

---

88 Dr. Steven Gundry, MD, *The Plant Paradox*, (Harper Wave; 1st edition, 2017), p. 282.

Vitamin C brings a wealth of health benefits. It contributes to the production and formation of collagen, helps wounds heal, strengthens bones and blood vessels, assists in iron absorption, is an antioxidant, and boosts your immune system. Like vitamin B, it is water-soluble, so daily supplementation is critical.

Figuring out how much vitamin C you need is easy. Just start with one tablet a day. (I like the brand EZ Melt because it dissolves in my mouth. I just think they're more effective, but there are lots of good brands on the market.) Wait a couple of days. As long as you don't experience any diarrhea, then you can add another one. Your body will tell you if you have had enough. If you start to experience loose stools, then go back to your previous dosage.

Magnesium

David has shared the challenge he's had over the years with regular bowel movements. If you're struggling to have a bowel movement every day, then I would suggest supplementing your meal plan with magnesium. We like Ancient Mineral Magnesium lotion because it's topical, which means it's not another supplement we're taking in pill form (there is no disadvantage to taking supplements as pills, it is just nice sometimes to have options.)

One pump a day of 20 mgs really helped David with his constipation. If that's not enough, you can always add a second pump a day. Magnesium is something that can be taken to bowel tolerance—meaning until the stools get too loose. You'll be able to tell within two to three days if it's helping. I've had clients report that it has helped them sleep better, improved skin irritations (apply directly to the irritated area), relieved sore muscles and helped with leg cramps and spasms. Magnesium is beneficial in so many ways; it's honestly one of my favorite supplements to add to everyone's regimen. There are many safe and effective options for magnesium supplements available on the market.

Blood Sugar Managers

I've seen great results in the management of some of my clients' glucose and hemoglobin A1c levels by adding a few supplements that they can get at Costco. One is called CinSulin, which combines chromium and cinnamon. Take two capsules a day. Then I suggest taking 30 mgs of zinc and 1,000 mgs of turmeric a day. This combination really helps them manage their blood sugar levels.

Reds, Greens, and Pre/Probiotics

There are three products we use and highly recommend that we buy from Dr. Gundry. I believe these are all foods/supplements that we can't get into our diets at the level we need for a variety of reasons. I like his products, and I trust their efficacy. Even though it gets expensive, I know if I tried to buy all these supplements separately, I'd pay a lot more for them. I also like that they are in powder form, so I can mix them up with water and drink them, which absorbs quickly since my body doesn't have to break them down. Here are the three we recommend for all our clients:

- **Vital Reds:** Dr. Gundry says that polyphenols might be the most important class of compounds missing from our diets. Polyphenols provide multiple benefits when metabolized by our gut bacteria. He formulated a one-of-a-kind blend that is loaded with thirty-four different polyphenols, plus his favorite probiotic.

- **Primal Plants:** You simply cannot eat enough greens in a day to get the benefits our guts need. There are a lot of greens-blend powders on the market, but most of them contain wheatgrass, barley grass, or oat grass, which can keep a leaky gut aggravated. Dr. Gundry's blend contains twelve superfood greens that are incredibly good for your gut and is gluten and lectin-free.
- **PrebioThrive:** Most people are familiar with probiotics. But do you know about prebiotics? Probiotics refer to the (healthy and necessary) bugs that live in and on us. Prebiotics are the compounds the probiotics need to eat. In essence, prebiotics feed the good guys while starving the bad guys in your gut. Dr. Gundry's prebiotic has all kinds of great foods for your gut microbiome that will help heal your leaky gut.

A Note about Swallowing Pills

Some people really struggle to take pills. If you are someone who has a hard time swallowing pills, there are still good options for you. If you buy supplements in capsule form, you can open them and mix the contents into a smoothie or other soft food. You can even do the same with pills; you just need to crush and then mix them into something else. Look into powders or lotions, or find a compounding pharmacy, where they may be able to customize your supplement as a liquid or topical. Please don't avoid supplementing with necessary nutrients if pill swallowing is the challenge. You may even find that you eventually become more comfortable with pills—just start with one pill at a time.

The list above provides an excellent starting point, but every body is unique. There may be other supplements your body needs in order to truly thrive and achieve optimal health. Every client I see is different, with different supplementation and dietary needs. We strongly encourage you to work with your doctor and find out which vitamins and minerals you are deficient in and add them to your daily routine.

It has truly made all the difference in our health journey. David and I eliminated the bad foods, and that made a big difference. We added good fats, lots of veggies, good sources of protein, fiber, and water, and we saw more improvement. Then we started supplementing our diets with the vitamins and minerals we were deficient in, and we felt a significant difference in energy levels, brain fog, and pain levels. We've become supplement converts!

When your body gets the nutrients it needs, it will reward you with improvement in so many areas of your health. Supplementing the proper foods with proper nutrition will help you to achieve your optimal health.

LIVING A PAIN-FREE LIFE

Jason McQuivey

I'd been in denial about my health for years. I have a stressful and sedentary job, and afternoon snacking and a late-night bowl of ice cream often got me through the day. It was hard to find time to exercise, plus I was so tired by the evening, it was the last thing I ever felt like doing. I didn't realize the toll it had taken on my body until I started experiencing some pretty severe back pain. The pain started in my lower back and would shoot down the back of my legs.

I went to chiropractors, massage therapists, and finally got an MRI. I was shocked when the doctor told me that, although I am just 51 years old, my back looks like that of a much older man. Sadly, surgery was likely in my future. I had cortisone shots in my spine that would help for a bit, but eventually the back pain would return. It got so bad that it kept me from participating in family activities and from being able to sleep.

One day, David Meine saw I was in obvious pain from the way I was walking. By that point, I'd seen many doctors, but David was the first person I'd met who could relate to what I was going through. He was also the first to suggest that the problem was probably related to inflammation caused by diet and lifestyle. He shared his story with me and urged me to read about Eating to Live. Desperate for relief, I immediately agreed and started working with Carla on Level 1.

It felt hard at first, but my body adjusted quickly, and it was so worth it as I started to feel better. I completely overhauled what I ate, eliminating all sugar and gluten. As someone who was used to lots of "meat and potatoes" meals (and let's be honest, lots of high-carb and processed foods as well), it was a lot of change. But I was committed; I was tired of living with constant pain! I tried to expand my horizons by adding a little fish and discovered I actually like poke! Carla and David encouraged me to continue to try to expand my palate and try new, healthy foods.

My constant back and leg pain almost disappeared. I started sleeping better. My energy levels increased dramatically. It's now been five weeks, and I've progressed to Level 2. I'm carefully journaling and tracking as I add foods, and it really is remarkable—if I slip up and have some gluten or sugar, the back pain returns. Originally, I wasn't sure the pain was linked to foods I was eating, but now the evidence has me convinced. Living without constant pain makes skipping my wife's chocolate cake or passing up on the deep-dish pizza worth it.

So far I've lost 20 pounds, but more importantly, I feel younger, happier, and more like myself than I have in years. I'm still a work in progress. I've got lots more to do to regain my health and have the quality of life I wish to live. But I refuse to age before my time any longer! I'm taking my life back by Eating to Live.

LEVEL 4

CHAPTER 1

AN INTRODUCTION TO LEVEL 4

Carla Meine

In Level 4 of the *Eating to Live* program, we focus on lifestyle choices that will help you to maintain the healthy choices you have recently been implementing in your life. Drawing on the power of your WHY, you've been motivated and self-disciplined with your food choices and daily journaling over the past weeks and months. You might want to take a moment and look through your journal to remember just how far you've come.

By the time you move into Level 4, you will likely be feeling significantly better than you did when you first started on this health journey. The steps you've taken to begin to heal your gut will likely be producing some wonderfully beneficial side effects by now. Hopefully, you're feeling an increase in energy during the day and sleeping better at night. Pain levels from inflammation in your body have probably decreased. As you've determined which foods your body can and cannot tolerate and eliminated those that cause problems for you, you should have less bloating, gas, or indigestion problems.

Level 4 is where we carefully reintroduce dairy into your diet. Like most of our clients, you're probably very excited to add some dairy back into your meal planning. Some of our clients can add all dairy products back with no problems at all. However, dairy is tricky. There is a reason it is the last food group we add back to our diets.

Adding dairy is typically the most challenging for our clients. For example, they might be able to add yogurt and hard cheeses and still be fine, but they don't tolerate other dairy products. Or perhaps they can add full heavy cream but struggle with milk of any kind. Some can handle cream cheese or sour cream but can't tolerate any ice cream at all. As you add dairy and continue to journal, you will discover which foods work for you.

Everyone is different. Your body will let you know which dairy products you can handle. By now, your leaky gut should be starting to heal as you are discovering all the foods that fuel your body and which foods you need to avoid.

Level 4 Meal Plan

In Level 4, you can continue to eat all of the foods your body tolerated well from Levels 1 through 3 as you carefully add dairy. Our clients love dairy, yet their bodies will end up telling them that it's struggling with it by having gas, bloating, constipation, etc. So, add it slowly. Add one item at a time, and wait a few days to see what happens before adding more.

Remember, you can always go back and take it out if you have too many issues. You're the scientist, and your body is the lab experiment. Track everything in your Eating to Live Journal to see which foods your body struggles with and which foods your body really likes. You are quickly becoming the expert on your body and what makes it feel its very best. This valuable information is what you will use as you continue on your journey to optimal health.

A Few Notes about Dairy Foods

Make sure you always choose pasture-raised and full-fat when you buy your dairy. We discussed the value of pasture-raised foods in previous levels, but for all of you who lived during the years of the "low-fat" craze and have spent your life buying skim milk, let me explain the truth we now know about full-fat dairy products.

There are many benefits—including weight loss. One reason for this is that fat is an incredibly satiating nutrient. It fills you up, so you're less likely to snack on other things. People who eat less fat tend to eat more refined carbs and sugar, which are the real problems for our health (and weight). Fat also slows the release of sugars into the bloodstream, which helps prevent overeating as well as blood sugar and insulin spikes in the body. Full-fat dairy is also lower in lactose, which is easier to digest than low-fat or no-fat products, and it helps raise healthy HDL cholesterol levels.

As you review the list of approved dairy foods below, you will notice that many of the items we recommend are probably different than the typical dairy that you've consumed in the past. You might be able to add some traditional dairy without issue, but most of the time, that's not the case. That's because cow's milk has both A2 and A1 beta-casein proteins, whereas milk from goats, sheep, and buffalo only has the A2, which is much easier for us to digest. Goat, sheep, and buffalo milks and cheeses are simply easier on our digestive systems than cow's milk and cheese.

Most of these items are readily available at health food stores. If your grocery store has a large deli section, you might be able to find them there as well. You can also order many of these products online.

Level 4

Vegetables	Peppers*	**Fruits**	**Seafood and Fish**	**Dairy Substitutes**
Arugula	Parsley	Apricots	Clams	Organic, full-fat coconut milk
Artichokes	Radicchio	Apples	Cod	Organic, un-sweetened nut milk
Asparagus	Radishes and leaves	Bananas	Crab	Almond milk
Avocado	Romaine lettuce	Blackberries	Halibut	Hazelnut milk
Acorn squash	Rutabaga	Blueberries	Herring	Hemp milk
Beets and beet greens	Scallions	Currants	Lobster	Yogurts made from coconut milk
Bok choy	Shallot	Cranberries	Mackerel	**Non-gluten Grains**
Beans, green	Squash	Cherries	Mussels	Almond four
Broccoli	Sweet potatoes	Dates	Oysters	Other nut flour

Brussel sprouts	Snow peas	Elderberries	Salmon	Amaranth
Bamboo shoots	Spinach	Figs	Sardines	Arrowroot
Chard	Seaweed	Grapes	Sea bass	Coconut flour
Chicory	Sea vegetable	Grapefruit	Shrimp	Cassava flour
Cilantro	Turnips and turnip greens	Goji berries	Trout	Flaxseeds/ flax
Collard greens	Tomatoes*	Honeydew melon	Tuna	Sorghum
Cabbage	Watercress	Kiwi	**Oils (cold-pressed)**	Tapioca
Celery	Water chestnuts	Lemon	Avocado oil	**Noodles**
Cucumber	Zucchini	Limes	Flax oil	Cappello's fettuccine
Carrots	Yams	Mango	Hemp oil	Pasta slim
Cauliflower	White potato (limit 1 per week)	Oranges	Olive oil (extra virgin)	Shirataki noodles
Chives	**Flavorings**	Pineapple	Nut oil	Kelp noodles
Dandelion greens	Coconut aminos	Pumpkin	MCT oil	Miracle noodles & Kanten pasta
Eggplant*	Herbs and spices	Pears	**Cooking Oils**	Miracle rice
Endive	Horseradish	Papaya	Avocado oil	Sweet potato noodles
Escarole	Himalayan sea salt	Peaches	Clarified butter/Ghee	Spaghetti squash noodles
Green peas (Green, split peas, black-eyed peas	Mustard	Plums	Coconut oil	Zucchini and squash noodles
Garlic	Nutritional yeast	Pomegranates	Pecan oil	Rice

Hearts of palm	Pickles	Passion fruit	Sesame oil	**Bone Broth**
Kale	Sauerkraut	Prunes	**Sweeteners** (1 tsp. per day)	1 cup per day, gluten-free, organic
Lettuce (all but iceberg)	Sea salt (preferably iodized)	Raspberries	Honey	**Beverages**
Leeks	Tamari (gluten-free only)	Rhubarb	Just Like Sugar	Water
Mushrooms	Wasabi (gluten-free only)	Raisins	Real maple syrup	Club soda
Mustard greens		Strawberries	Molasses	Coffee (limit 2 cups per day)
Mizuna		Tangerines	Monk fruit	Tea (black, green, white, red root, oolong, match, herbal)
Onions		Watermelon	Sorghum	Yerba mate
Okra		**Vinegars**	Stevia	Kombucha tea
Olives		Any, if no added sugar	Swerve	**Chocolate**
			Xylitol	70% or greater, 1 oz. per day
Poultry**	Eggs** (pasture-raised only)	**Nuts & Seeds**** (if you can tolerate them)	**Meats***** (grass-fed, humanely-raised, or wild when possible)	

Chicken	Chicken	Tree Nuts • Almonds • Walnuts • Hazelnuts • Cashews • Brazil nuts • Pistachios • Macadamia nuts • Pecans • Chestnuts • Pinenuts	Beef	**Dairy****** (always choose pasture-raised and full-fat)
Duck	Duck	Seeds • Sunflower • Pumpkin • Sesame • Flax • Chia • Psyllium	Bison	Butter (pasture-raised, Italian, or French)
Dove		Peanuts	Brain	Buffalo butter
Goose		Tahini	Elk	Cream cheese (organic)
Pheasant		Sunflower butter	Gizzard	French/ Italian cheese
Turkey		Almond butter	Heart	Ghee
			Kidney	Goat yogurt
			Liver	Goat cheese
			Lamb	Goat or sheep kefir
			Pork	Heavy cream (organic)
			Sweet breads	Milk (casein A2, if possible)
			Tongue	Sheep cheese and yogurt

			Veal	Sour cream (organic)
			Venison	Mozzarella (buffalo, if available)
				Parmigiano-Reggiano
				Whey protein powder

**unless you have issues*
***Level 2 food group additions*
****Level 3 food group additions*
*****Level 4 food group additions*

CHAPTER 2

REDUCE STRESS

David Meine

Throughout the course of my life, I've had almost unlimited opportunities to learn about stress. Consider this stressful moment that happened a few years ago when I was battling extreme pain from foot neuropathy:

"Carla, I cannot believe it—the medication for my neuropathy is going to cost us $700 per month, out of pocket, because of our crummy health insurance!" I lamented to my wife as I read the pharmacy receipt. "Plus, since it's a controlled substance, I can't get more than a thirty-day supply!" Carla could tell I was getting wound up and shook her head sympathetically. My mind was churning at a million miles per hour, and I could feel my heart rate increasing.

I reminded myself that I knew what to do to calm myself down, and mentally I pushed pause. I took a deep breath and held it for the count of three. Then I opened my mouth and slowly exhaled. After breathing normally for twenty seconds, I took another deep breath and repeated the sequence twice more. I felt calmer and more in control of my emotions after I finished this simple stress-reducing exercise.

We live in a stressful world. Stress comes in all shapes and sizes. We can experience financial stress, familial stress, job stress—it can feel like a pretty long list! Our bodies are actually fairly well-equipped to handle stress in small doses, but when we are pounded by stressors again and again in chronic or long-term situations, it has serious effects on our health. In fact, stress affects all of our body's systems, including musculoskeletal, respiratory, cardiovascular, endocrine, gastrointestinal, nervous, and reproductive systems.[89] Stress that's left unchecked contributes to many health problems, like high blood pressure, heart disease, obesity, and diabetes. And we all know, we just feel super crappy when we're stressed out.

Stress isn't all bad. For example, stress helps us to be motivated and rise to meet challenges. It can help us to work more efficiently. It also serves as a vital warning system. But once we start experiencing stress in unhealthy ways, a very vicious cycle can start. We tend to eat too much of the wrong foods, which increases the stress on our bodies. When we're stressed, we often drink unhealthy beverages, which dramatically increase poor brain function. These behaviors all lead to poor sleep that keeps us from experiencing the REM and deep sleep necessary to repair the body.

On top of all this, stress greatly affects the gut. Remember that brain-gut connection we discussed earlier? The gut is inhabited

---

89 "Stress effects on the body," American Psychological Association, 1 November, 2018, *https://www.apa.org/topics/stress/body.*

by millions of bacteria, and those bacteria are affected by stress. This means that our gut microbiome, which is so essential to our health, is altered when we are experiencing stress. This affects the health of our brain *and* our body and opens the door to problems like leaky gut syndrome, which further diminishes our immune system and creates inflammation that is so detrimental to our bodies. If you have inflammation throughout your body and your brain, it is pretty challenging to manage stress well.

So how can we keep stress in check when life tends to be pretty stressful? The first step in effective stress management is recognizing the negative symptoms in real-time and having some techniques in your arsenal to manage them on the spot. There are also things we can do to prevent or manage stress in the long run. Here are seven simple ways to reduce and manage stress.

1. **Mindful Meditation and Visualization Exercises**
   "Meditation" and "visualization" are more than buzzwords. They are straightforward, easy-to-access techniques for managing stress. The mental and physical health benefits they offer are extensive, and they're also thoroughly backed by science. In a study conducted by Harvard Medical School, subjects who participated in an eight-week meditation program actually showed an increase in gray matter in the parts of the brain responsible for learning, memory, and emotional regulation.[90]

---

90 Erin Heger, "7 benefits of meditation, and how it can affect your brain," Insider, 19 May 2020, *https://www.insider.com/benefits-of-meditation.*

Mindfulness meditation is a mental-training practice that helps calm both your body and mind. It helps train your mind to focus on the present and to eliminate that pesky overthinking and ruminating we do that fuels anxiety. Regular practitioners have lower levels of cortisol—the stress hormone that we'll discuss more below—and report lower levels of burnout. Mindful meditation and visualization can also help with trouble sleeping, loss of appetite due to stress, and depression. I have utilized mindfulness meditation and visualization techniques for many years. They have helped me as I've fought to control pain due to various health issues, as well as the stress in my life. After studying the science of brain training for many years, I've developed courses to help clients lose weight, sleep better, and relax. I know these techniques are powerful and positive ways we can better manage high levels of stress, and they can be game-changers on our journey to optimal health.

At *Eating to Live*, we have created some specialized visualization exercises to help you learn to focus as you employ helpful relaxation techniques. These techniques will allow you to decrease negative stress and help combat inflammation in the brain and body. You can find these at *www.eatingtolive.com/book*.

2. **Exercise**

In the next chapter, Carla and I will discuss how critical exercise is for optimal health. But here are just a few reasons that it is so helpful in managing stress.

Exercise lowers the body's stress hormones. Cortisol, an important steroid hormone that regulates many processes throughout the body, plays an important role in helping the body respond to stress. But it wreaks havoc in the body when there is too much of it. Overexposure to cortisol and other stress hormones disrupts almost all of your body's processes.

When you feel well, it is easier to handle stress and manage cortisol levels. Exercise releases endorphins, which are chemicals that improve mood and act as natural painkillers. Exercise promotes confidence when done regularly, and this confidence fosters a sense of wellbeing.

Stress is a major disruptor of sleep. Regular exercise can help us to sleep better, which is so foundational to achieving optimal health.

3. **Laughter**

   Did you know that it's been scientifically proven that laughing reduces stress? A recent study of rural Midwestern cancer patients revealed that humor has amazing benefits. In this study, thirty-three patients were shown videos. One group watched tourism videos, while the other group watched funny videos.

   The results showed that the group who laughed as they watched funny videos not only had lower levels of stress, but they also had increased immune function! The study concluded that due to such marked improvement in immune system cell activity, laughter could be considered a helpful cognitive-behavior intervention for both health and stress management.[91]

   Look for humor and find ways to laugh, even when you're feeling extra stress in your life. Watch your favorite funny movies (*The Princess Bride* is one of my

---

91 Mary P. Bennett, et al., "The effect of mirthful laughter on stress and natural killer cell activity," Pubmed.gov, March-April 2003, https://pubmed.ncbi.nlm.nih.gov/12652882/.

go-tos; there are so many good one-liners that make me laugh every time!). Watching or listening to something funny can provide an instant lift in life.

Find positive people who make you laugh and try to spend more time with them. You can also choose to *be* one of those people. I grew up with a lot of adversity and can remember consciously realizing that I had to choose between being grouchy and moody or happy and funny, no matter what life threw at me. I've learned that people with a cheerful disposition attract positive people and experiences in their life. I want to be one of those people!

Lastly, be sure to laugh at yourself! Over the years, Carla has taught me not to make jokes at others' expenses. She says it is always better to make fun of myself or a personal situation to get a laugh. I have found there is plenty to laugh about, and it helps me not take myself too seriously. I am convinced that laughter has helped improve my health and mental wellbeing.

4. **Seriously Consider Supplements**

   Have you ever asked yourself how vitamin and mineral deficiencies contribute to stress? I'm always surprised that these deficiencies are typically not considered when someone is diagnosed with some form of depression. Why is diet not evaluated to determine if there are essential vitamin and mineral deficits?

   Until I invested in myself by having a blood analysis done, I never really knew what my brain and body lacked in order to operate at optimal performance. Someday, I hope there will be a device that can give us a simple blood scan with results delivered instantaneously, like what Dr. McCoy uses on *Star Trek*. Until that becomes a reality, I encourage you to invest in your own health and see what your body is lacking.

We've already talked about supplements, but there are two in particular that can help combat stress: omega 3s and B complex vitamins. Taking a B complex can help relieve stress and keep your energy high.[92] In a study conducted over thirty years, scientists found that omega-3s reduce both anxiety and inflammation.[93] I also recommend taking magnesium (we prefer it as a topical; refer to the chapter on supplements in Level 3), as it combats insomnia, a frequent side effect of stress. Adding 500 mgs a day has shown to increase sleep time, improve sleep efficiency, and help you fall asleep faster.[94]

Reviewing my year-over-year lab work for the past three years has proven that taking supplements daily dramatically and positively affected my health. Adding the right supplements to the right diet has given me a fantastic quality of life.

Note: Some supplements can interact with medications or have side effects, so you should consult with a doctor if

---

92 Con Stough, et al., "Reducing occupational stress with a B-vitamin focussed intervention: a randomized clinical trial: study protocol," US National Library of Medicine and National Institutes of Health, 22 December 2014, *https://www.ncbi.nlm.nih.gov/pmc/articles/PMC4290459/.*

93 Grace Rattue, "OMEGA-3 Has Beneficial Effect On Anxiety And Inflammation," Medical News Today, 11 November 2011, *https://www.medicalnewstoday.com/articles/237508#1.*

94 Behnood Abbasi, et al., "The effect of magnesium supplementation on primary insomnia in elderly: A double-blind placebo-controlled clinical trial," Pubmed.gov, December 2012, *https://pubmed.ncbi.nlm.nih.gov/23853635/.*

you have a medical condition. Please read all labels when evaluating supplements.

5. **Reach Out to Others**

Human connection is so vital to our health. If we want to live longer and healthier lives, we need to stay connected to others in our community. We live in an age of ever-increasing loneliness and social isolation. Researchers warn that loneliness can be as damaging to health as smoking fifteen cigarettes a day![95] Loneliness has been found to increase cortisol and inflammation levels, and it definitely makes combating stress much more difficult.

The good news is that research also proves people with healthy and supportive relationships live longer and healthier lives. Taking the time to connect with others activates beneficial processes in our bodies, specifically the release of oxytocin. Oxytocin reduces cortisol and pain, and it actually changes the way our brain responds to potential stressors. It even promotes the growth of new brain cells! Hugs increase natural oxytocin levels, as does eye contact. Even making eye contact with your dog increases oxytocin![96] We release oxytocin when taking care of children or spending time with friends. This is called the "tend and befriend effect," and it's the

95 "The Loneliness Epidemic," Health Resources & Service Administration (HRSA), January 2019, *https://www.hrsa.gov/enews/past-issues/2019/january-17/loneliness-epidemic.*

96 Elizabeth Hopper, "How Your Social Life Might Help You Live Longer," Greater Good Magazine, 28 July 2020, *https://greatergood.berkeley.edu/article/item/how_your_social_life_might_help_you_life_longer.*

opposite of the flight-or-fight response generated by stress.[97]

Some people have built-in relationships they can access for this kind of support. Others may find themselves wondering how to improve relationships and connections with others. If this is you, here are some easy ways to turn outward and increase the amount of connection you have in your life:

- Volunteer. Find an organization or cause that needs help. You won't have to look far to find something, I promise! Studies show that those who volunteer tend to live longer—the kind of benefit usually received from eating lots of fruits and vegetables. Elderly people who volunteered regularly were 44% less likely to die over the course of a five-year study. Volunteers also show lower levels of measurable inflammation in their systems.
- Perform random acts of kindness. Find little things you can do as you go about your day that make someone else feel good. Talk to the person behind you in line at the grocery checkout. Smile and make eye contact with your neighbor when you get your mail. Take someone's garbage cans back in for them, even if they didn't ask. Research suggests those who engage in "kind acts" have changes in their immune system genes that help wellbeing and longevity.
- Call someone. Catching up with someone helps our health. A phone call is better than texting, as more

97 S. E. Taylor, et al., "Biobehavioral responses to stress in females: tend-and-befriend, not fight-or-flight," National Library of Medicine, July 2000, *https://pubmed.ncbi.nlm.nih.gov/10941275/.*

oxytocin is released from talking on the phone than having the same conversation over text.[98]

If you are someone who has some built-in relationships you can rely on, don't take them for granted! Make sure you're finding opportunities to strengthen those relationships and stay connected. Take your spouse or partner on a date. Have a family game night. Ask a friend how they're doing and initiate a good conversation. If you feel stressed right now, pick up the phone and reach out to one of them.

I am so grateful for my family and network of friends. Being able to communicate with someone I trust, someone who goes through the happy and the hard times with me, helps me lower my physical and mental stress. Inevitably, having a nonjudgmental listening ear always helps me feel better. Maintaining these relationships takes effort, but it's so important. Just like we take the time to meal plan for healthy eating or train to run a 5K, spending quality time with friends and family is equally important to your health and wellbeing.

6. **Reduce Your Intake of Caffeine**

   By now, you've already heard me talk about the negative effects of caffeine as related to our health and getting quality sleep. But caffeine can also cause increased levels of anxiety. Individuals have different threshold levels for how much caffeine they can tolerate. If you notice that you tend to be stressed, jittery, or anxious,

98 Elizabeth Hopper, "How Your Social Life Might Help You Live Longer," Greater Good Magazine, 28 July 2020, *https://greatergood.berkeley.edu/article/item/how_your_social_life_might_help_you_life_longer.*

please seriously consider cutting back on your caffeine intake.

If you are a regular consumer of caffeine, try this experiment: Commit to eliminating caffeine for one week. The first few days might be hard as you experience withdrawal symptoms, which simply means you have a problem that is worth fixing to improve your health. But after that, journal each day. Write down how you feel. Record your levels of stress. Use a simple rating scale of one to five and rank your anxiety levels. I want you to create an opportunity for you to be a scientist. It's all about cause and effect.

We believe in taking small steps to get on the right track for achieving optimal health. Cutting back on caffeine can be a really important step in the right direction on your health journey.

7. **Journaling Gratitude**

   When we get stressed, it's so easy to focus on the negative. Remembering to be grateful for the good things in our life helps to lower stress. Counting our blessings is scientifically proven to help both our health and our happiness. Developing an attitude of gratitude is much easier if you can find time to journal your life's positive aspects. Studies say there are significant benefits from journaling a mere fifteen minutes, three times a week, in a gratitude journal.[99]

   I am striving to be consistent at gratitude journaling. I've recently learned more about the science behind effective gratitude journaling and have modified what I write each week.

---

99 Greater Good in Action, *https://ggia.berkeley.edu/practice/gratitude_journal.*

Focusing on people for whom you are grateful has more of an impact than focusing on things, so the majority of my gratitude journaling is now focused on the people in my life. Studies also say to be specific about what I'm grateful for. So instead of writing, "I'm so grateful for Sam," I write, "I'm so grateful that Sam took the time to go fishing with me yesterday."

Here is a fascinating insight: When I get upset or stressed with someone who I have previously written about in my gratitude journal, I immediately start to think about the positive ways they have affected me. This thought process softens my feelings about them and, in turn, begins to diminish my stress dramatically.

In short, the practice of gratitude is something that takes little effort while yielding high results in helping us manage feelings of stress and anxiety in our life.

These are just a few ideas to decrease stress; there are many others you can explore and employ. Here are just a few more:

- Listening to soothing music
- Using essential oils
- Getting massages
- Practicing a hobby that you love
- Getting out in nature

Find what works for you!

The Bottom Line

Stress and anxiety can be helpful to grow and succeed in certain situations. But when pressures cross the boundary of healthy tolerance, it's necessary to do something to get your mind away from the source of the stress. Find what works for you. Practice both preventative and "emergency, in-the-moment" stress management techniques. Effective stress management will help you immensely as you work to achieve your optimal health.

CHAPTER 3

EXERCISE FOR A HEALTHY BODY

David and Carla Meine

"If you don't make time for exercise, you'll probably have to make time for illness."

—ROBIN SHARMA

David: His Perspective

I am so grateful that I have learned the personal benefits that exercise gives me. Counting reps puts me in my happy place as I release endorphins. Exercise therapy works my body's two most important organs. The first and most critical organ that benefits from this therapy is my brain. The second critical organ is my heart.

It might surprise you that the brain benefits so much from exercise, but it's true. I have been so frustrated by brain fog and my memory issues over the years. Exercise played a key role in improving my brain's performance.

Exercise increases your heart rate, which pumps more oxygen to the brain. The hormones that are released in your brain provide an optimum environment for brain cell growth and promote brain plasticity. Research even shows that exercise increases growth factors in the brain, which makes it easier for the brain to grow new neuronal connections.[100]

In addition to helping the brain function better, exercising also affects the brain in ways that make you feel better. A *lot* better! That's because when you exercise, your body releases dopamine and endorphins in your brain. These are the "feel-good" chemicals that make you happy. Exercise also helps your brain to eliminate chemicals that make you feel stressed or anxious. I'd call that a win-win-win.

Carla: Her Perspective

Something I hear a lot is, "It must be so easy for you to stay healthy. You seem to love to exercise. It is so difficult for me!" The truth of it is that almost every day, I have to talk myself into getting up and doing my exercise routine. So many mornings, I just want to skip it and stay in bed a little longer. So I lay there having a conversation with myself that goes something like this:

"I think I'll just skip my workout today."

"You know you'll be sorry if you do. You always feel better after you're done."

---

100 Brock Armstrong, "How Exercise Affects Your Brain," Scientific American, 6 December 2018, *https://www.scientificamerican.com/article/how-exercise-affects-your-brain/.*

"I know, but missing just today won't matter that much. It's fine!"

"You know that if you skip today, it will get easier to skip tomorrow."

"I know, but I just don't feel like it today."

"You know if you get up right now and go get it done, you're going to feel so much better than you do right now. So if you want to feel better, just go get your workout done."

"Alright, alright, I'll get it done just for today."

Is that the kind of conversation someone who seems to love to exercise would repeatedly have with themselves? Yet, I have this talk with myself several times a week. One thing that helps me to get up and do it is that I never regret the choice to exercise. There are lots of other choices I could make that I might regret, but I never finish a workout and wish I'd done something else instead.

David: Self-Care

One of my favorite ways to work out is by using online cycling trainers on my NordicTrack® iFit® 22i Series bike. These trainers frequently mention a concept called "self-care." I want to be better at this for myself and to help motivate others to engage in their own self-care in order to achieve their optimal health.

Self-care includes (but is not limited to) many of the healthy lifestyle choices we have discussed in this book. Sadly, we live in a modern, demanding world where self-care is challenging. Finding time in our busy schedules can be overwhelming. It requires effort and discipline. Some of us might even feel guilty when we think about putting ourselves and our own needs before the needs of others. But I believe that, in our heart of hearts, we know taking good care of ourselves is the very best thing we can do for those we love.

I also believe that the quote we shared from Robin Sharma at the beginning of this chapter is so true. And we like to expand it to include all aspects of healthy living and self-care.

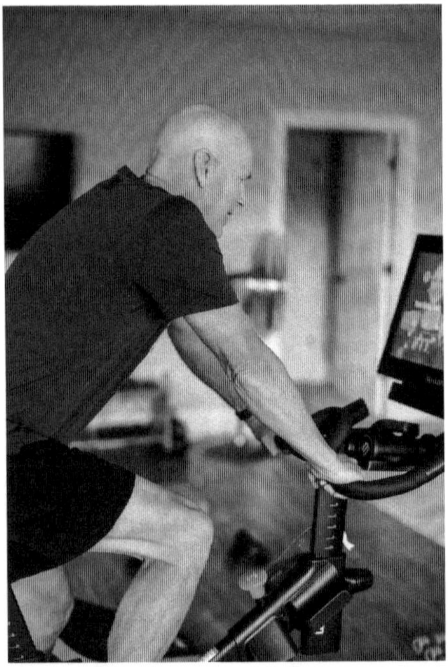

If we don't make time to take care of ourselves—through proper diet, exercise, sleep, and other aspects of self-care—we will likely have to make time for illness and other problems down the road.

From the first half of this book, you've seen that I've had more than my fair share of illnesses. It took me a long time and a lot of hard work to figure out how much I needed to change about my diet so that I could heal my leaky gut and enjoy a pain-free, healthy life. Exercise and fat loss have been an important part of this journey.

It was such a wake-up call when I learned I was yoked with 5.29 pounds (2.4 kgs) of visceral fat wrapped around my organs. This really made me reevaluate my exercise routine. Studying how to get rid of visceral fat has been encouraging.

The image below shows what it looks like to have visceral fat versus subcutaneous fat. I have been working hard to eliminate the threat this fat poses to me and to look like the "standard type" in the middle. I am trying to get my visceral fat to below one pound, which will have an important effect on my optimal health. Working with this goal in mind has helped strengthen my WHY and kept me motivated in my exercise goals.

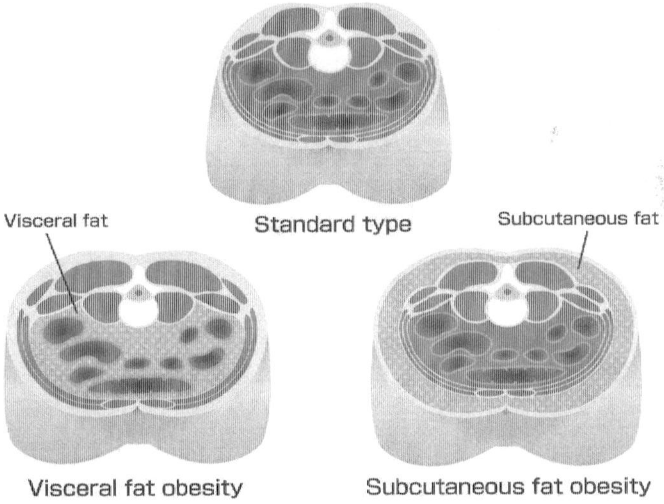

Carla: What Works for Me

At *Eating to Live*, we recommend at least thirty minutes of exercise, five days a week. People often ask what I do, which is typically thirty to sixty minutes of exercise six days a week

(I always take Sundays off and give my body a rest, which is extremely important). So, what do I do to make sure I do it, even on the days I don't feel like doing it?

I do things like set up times to meet my friends in the morning for a brisk walk. When I know someone else will be there waiting for me to walk with them, it motivates me to get up and show up. I also set up pickleball games (if you haven't heard of this fun sport, you need to search it on YouTube) to play later in the week. That way, when the day comes, and I'm not feeling up to playing, once again, I know there are three other people counting on me to be there. Plus, if you're socializing as you're working out, you're getting twice the bang for your workout buck!

On the days I don't have plans with others, I have a workout routine I do in my basement with a few weights. I set a goal to do this twenty-minute core workout three days a week. I set another goal to cycle for thirty minutes three days a week. Goals are an important part of following through on exercise each day.

Being able to measure positive results of meeting these goals is very rewarding. According to my body scan, I've put on four pounds of muscle this past year doing this. I think that's pretty good at sixty-two years old! My new goal is to put on another four pounds of muscle next year. I'm really motivated to achieve this goal, and it helps me stick to the exercise goals I've set for myself.

Another thing I suggest to my clients is to start slow and not overdo it. Nothing kills a desire to improve like an injury. If you've done nothing for years, start by just getting out and walking around the block. Then add another block. Keep slowly adding distance until you can walk for thirty minutes. Many of us live near a mall. In the winter, walking the mall is a great option. Take a friend and have a fun conversation, and the time passes so quickly! If you find it motivating, perhaps you want to get a watch that counts steps. My good friend's eighty-two-year-old mother has lost over fifty pounds by meeting (and very often exceeding!) her goal of 10,000 steps a day. No matter what, she gets in those steps!

If you've never done a workout routine before, then start with simple exercises just using your own body weight. Do a few squats, sit-ups, and push-ups to start. There are lots of free videos online that you can follow. Who knows? Maybe if you follow us on social media, we'll do a few of them too. Again, start slow, and just work your way up.

What's most important is to find something that you like to do. If you absolutely hate running, don't run! Maybe Zumba class is a better fit for you. Find a fun sport or activity that you like to do. Sometimes you need to do several of them to figure out what works for you. I have a son who likes to hike, so I plan a hike with him every couple of weeks. This way, I'm committed to a workout, and it's great one-on-one time with him in the mountains. Currently, I like pickleball, but years ago it was tennis. I love to cycle, so I try to incorporate that into my workouts. I really enjoy time with friends and family, so they are a big part of my workout routine. Find something and someone who helps you start and stay motivated.

Eventually, you'll discover that the way you feel after a workout is part of the motivation as well. As your mind, heart, and body grow stronger, you'll feel better physically, mentally, and emotionally. You'll have increased energy and likely even sleep better at night. And, you'll be well on your way to achieving your optimal health.

David: What Works for Me

I have always had to have a strong WHY statement/goal to stay motivated to exercise. At my age, and because of some prior injuries, I have become limited in the type of activities I can do for exercise. For example, the best way to lose visceral fat is aerobic exercise. Those include swimming, cycling, running, and basically any activity that gets the heart pumping. This heart-pumping exercise needs to maintain a high heart rate for an extended period of time. I try to find activities that aren't so hard on my body. Recently, I discovered pool cardio, which provides excellent muscle resistance while not being hard on tendons and joints.

As Carla said, it's most important that you find something you enjoy doing. Then, make a goal to do it thirty to sixty minutes a day, three to five days a week.

Here is an example of my exercise routine when I am home:

- **Monday:** 30 to 60 minutes of indoor or outdoor cycling, based on weather conditions.
- **Tuesday:** 20 minutes of core exercise and resistance exercises; 30 minutes of walking indoors or outdoors, based on weather conditions.
- **Wednesday:** 45 easy minutes of indoor or outdoor cycling, based on weather conditions.

- **Thursday:** 20 minutes of core exercise and resistance exercises; 30 minutes of walking indoors or outdoors, based on weather conditions.
- **Friday:** Fishing for hours up and down a river.
- **Saturday:** 2-hour bike ride, weather permitting, or 30 to 60 minutes of high-intensity indoor cycling.
- **Sunday:** Rest and recovery day.

When I am traveling, I try to fit exercise in as well. If the weather permits, I walk three miles a day. Sometimes, I find a mall I can walk in when I travel. If I am staying at a hotel with an exercise room, I try to do some resistance training for thirty minutes every other day. Sunday is always a rest and recovery day.

Some Additional Fun Workout Ideas that Work for Me

At home, as part of my resistance training, I use a core training exercise device called a Stealth Trainer. This turns exercise into a fun game. You download the app and put your mobile phone on the trainer. While balancing on the board with your core engaged, you move the board back and forth to line up exploding game dots on your phone screen. I like how it keeps me distracted and engaged while I do three sets.

For years, I have used a simple push-up device called the Perfect Pushup®. Invented by a US Navy SEAL to optimize the basic push-up, the Perfect Fitness Perfect Pushup reduces pressure on the hands and wrists while increasing strength and definition in arms, shoulders, chest, back, and core. I keep this as a regular part of my exercise routine based on its simplicity, and it keeps me from getting injuries.

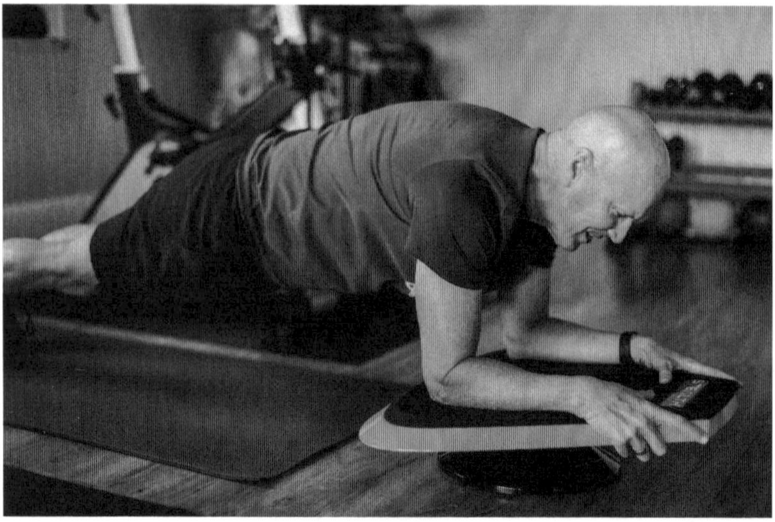

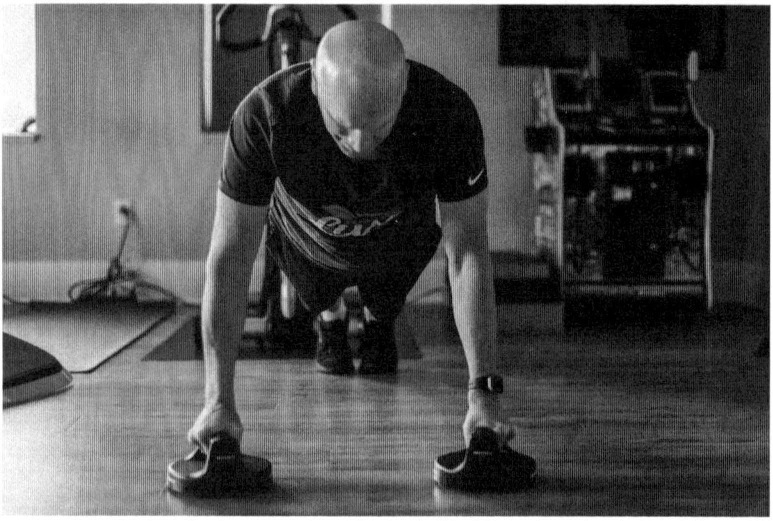

Consuming quality calories, getting quality sleep, drinking enough water, and exercising regularly make up the four pillars of health. Since my cancer battle in 2015, I have focused on these four pillars. Exercise is definitely the most difficult of the four to maintain. We can't function without water, food, and sleep. But we can go for years without exercising...perhaps until it's too late.

It takes a strong WHY to develop the discipline necessary to exercise consistently. But it is impossible to live a healthy life without it. We only get one body! It is so important to keep it healthy by getting up and getting that blood pumping. I find that when I consistently exercise, I don't need sugar, caffeine, or any other drug to get those feel-good hormones.

The famous Charlie Chaplin once said, "The six best doctors in the world are the sun, rest, exercise, diet, self-respect, and friends. Stick to them at all stages of your life and enjoy a healthy life..."[101] I agree and maintain that, through exercise, you can capitalize on all six at once!

Your Journey to Optimal Health

We are at the end of this narrative, but it's certainly not the end of the journey. Take a moment and think about where you are on your own journey to optimal health. For some of you, this might be a courageous new beginning. Others might have already started on the road to health but need a little "rerouting." For so long, I lived what I thought was a healthy lifestyle, yet my problems persisted, and the ailments increased. Getting it right required quite a bit of rerouting for me.

As you look at your life, ask yourself, is your health where you want it to be? Do you have the energy and vitality you need to

---

101 Larry Slabotsky, "Charlie Chaplin's 4 Life Rules," Retire to 100, 1 March 2021, *https://www.retireto100.com/posts/2021/3/1/charlie-chaplins-4-life-rules.*

get through the day? Have you been ignoring some pain and discomfort or perhaps treating those symptoms instead of their root causes? There are definitely some health conditions we cannot cure or control on our own, but there is *so very much within our control.*

Even small changes made over a long period of time are so beneficial. And, small changes are actually more doable than trying to change everything at once, only to throw in the towel when it gets hard. If you're thinking it's time to make some changes in your life, pick one that's important to you and build from there. Today is the oldest you have ever been and the youngest you will ever be. The good news is that it's not too late! You can start today.

We only get one shot at this thing called life. And we only get one body for the journey. As someone once said, "The idea is to die young as late as possible."[102] It's possible as we begin to access a life of health, vitality, and wellness. It's possible as we start healing our guts, making healthy lifestyle choices, and eating to live. It's possible to not only survive but to thrive and to live your very best life.

---

102 "Ashley Montagu Quotes and Sayings - Page 1," inspiringquotes.us, *https://www.inspiringquotes.us/author/4575-ashley-montagu.*

CONCLUSION

EPILOGUE

May 3, 2021

I am often asked, "How are you doing, David?" Caring friends and family who know about my years of health challenges want to know how it's all going. I love answering that question now. I get the biggest smile on my face and tell them I feel absolutely amazing! And each and every time I say it, I am thankful for the quality of life that I am enjoying. It feels like a miracle—a gift.

Gratefully, I am still in remission from my bladder cancer. I have no back pain, which had been so debilitating for me for years. I no longer deal with stomach bloating, constipation, arthritis, heartburn, erectile dysfunction, or that miserable peripheral neuropathy. I rarely get seasonally sick with colds or flus, especially considering how frequently I did the first sixty-three years of my life. And compared to my friends, I have far fewer of the typical old-age aches and pains, and they're all envious of my newfound energy levels.

And, I'm no longer juggling multiple prescription medications and fretting about their unwelcome side effects. That's right—I'm off of every single prescription! When I started this journey, I was taking five. I'm down to zero. I'm also off every over-the-counter medicine I used to rely so heavily on; no more Tums, Pepto Bismol, melatonin, and no more NSAIDs! It took commitment and hard work, but wow, it was worth it.

A very surprising side effect is that, through cutting out sugar, gluten, and other foods my gut is sensitive to, my body has "right-sized." So, although I wasn't on a journey to lose weight and was fairly comfortable at the 204 pounds I used to sit at, I'm now right around 185 pounds. This has helped my pickleball game and my cycling, and it all feels really good!

Perhaps the best part, though, is that my pervasive brain fog and memory issues have completely disappeared. I could shout for joy about this one benefit alone. Carla tells everyone that I now have a better memory than she does. What a compliment! I'm so happy to be operating at "full capacity" again.

I remain amazed that my overall daily pain level is typically zero. Just three years ago, I was suffering immensely, even while taking multiple medications every day for pain. This is miraculous to me. When I share my story with people, they look at me in disbelief. You might be thinking that the word "miracle" is hyperbole. But to me—and to Carla, who has watched me suffer and struggle and been there with me for every step of the way—"miracle" remains the only appropriate vocabulary choice.

Thanks are due to my dream team of doctors. The path to healing started with Dr. Khan and continued with Dr. Gundry and Dr. O'Bryan. I could not have done any of it without my dear wife, Carla, who is now blessing many others with her immense knowledge and experience as a Certified Functional Nutrition Counselor.

Every time I follow up with my doctors, the results are impressive. In January of 2021, we met again with Dr. Gundry to review my labs. Before the appointment, I worried that the results wouldn't be as good as I'd hoped. But I needn't have stressed; all my efforts were paying off. Here are just a few highlights from our discussion:

- My IL-16 score, which deals with Acute Coronary Syndrome (ACS) and measures my potential for a heart attack compared to men my same age, had dropped. What a relief it was to see this positive result after being so despondent about these results in years past.
- The score indicative of leaky gut had been cut in half from the previous year. I now had proof that my gut was healing!
- My vitamin D levels, which had been so low in my first lab reports in 2018, were now at a very healthy 147. Dr. Gundry shared some interesting studies happening at UC San Diego showing that people who get cancer have low vitamin D. People with high vitamin D have far less cancer in their medical histories. We were especially happy with this news, as we are trying to keep me in remission with my bladder cancer.
- Dr. Gundry was excited that my triglyceride score was 82. My scores in 2018 and 2020 were 147 and 143, respectively, so this was a significant improvement. He then rained on my parade a bit when he told me that

> he'd like me to get down to a 40 or 50, but at least I'm definitely headed in the right direction.

After reviewing these and many other positive results of my blood work, I asked Dr. Gundry one last question. "I have one final medication to get off of," I said. "I'd like to be able to get off Finasteride for my enlarged prostate." This condition, which affects over 50% of men ages fifty-one and older, kept me chained to this one last prescription medication, and I wanted to be free of it.

He explained that high insulin levels stimulate this prostate condition. My insulin level at the time was a 7.5, and he wanted me to be at a six. I'd been improving year over year. "You're on the right track, David," he encouraged. "You've got to be very diligent about staying away from sugars and starches. If you stay the course, I think you'll be able to stop taking Finasteride." I stayed the course, and he was right. I am free from all prescription medications!

Carla had her appointment after mine, and she was very pleased with all of her results as well. We left Dr. Gundry's office with huge smiles on our faces, feeling on top of the world.

The journey over the past three years (and all of those years of struggle before that) has been bumpy and long. The path has not been straight or easy. There have been many twists and turns on this journey. But, all journeys start with a small step. The first step for me was being open-minded to what I was learning. The next step was believing that *I could do it*; I really did have the power to take back my health and lower my risk of future health problems. Many more small steps followed as both Carla and I persevered. We persisted. And then we started seeing the results, and even more importantly, *feeling* the results, and suddenly, every hard step along the way was incredibly, absolutely worth it.

We hope you'll join us on this journey to health and wellbeing. You can see what we're doing at www.eatingtolive.com, where we're constantly creating new resources and tools for overcoming leaky gut and other health challenges. It is our hope that we can help others improve their quality of life and start their own journey to achieving optimal health.

Thank you for letting us share our story with you.

Carla and David Meine

APPENDIX I

1. Post-Sleep Questionnaire
2. Sleep Study Results Form
3. PULS Cardiac Test
4. Salveo Diagnostics Report
5. Veridia Diagnostics Report
6. True Health Diagnostics
7. Supplements Page
8. PULS Report #2
9. Quest Diagnostics Report
10. Supplements Page #2
11. Dexa Body Scan Report

1. Post-Sleep Questionnaire

Revere Health

Sleep Disorders Center

Name: David Meine

Date: 11/29/17

Post-sleep Questionnaire

1. How long do you feel it took you to fall asleep? Few minutes
   How does this compare to your "normal"?
   Longer than normal _____ About normal ✓ Shorter than normal _____
2. How many hours do you feel you slept last night? 7 hours
   How does this compare to a "normal" night at home?
   Longer than normal _____ About normal ✓ Shorter than normal _____
3. Do you remember waking up during the night? Yes ✓ No _____
   If yes, how many times? 2 Did it take long to fall back asleep Yes ____ No ✓
4. How would you rate the quality of your sleep?
   Bad _____ Poor ✓ Fair | Good _____ Excellent _____
   How does this compare to a "normal" night at home? Worse ✓ Same ___ Better ___
5. Do you remember dreaming during the night? Yes _____ No ✓
6. Will you be driving yourself home this morning? Yes ✓ No _____
   If yes, do you feel awake and alert enough to drive this morning? Yes ✓ No _____
   If no, is there someone we can call to pick you up and drive you home?
   Name: __________ Phone: __________
7. Do you feel the tech educated you well on what was happening?
   Yes
8. If you were tried on CPAP, were you measured and given the option for multiple masks?
   NO
9. How would you rate the quality of service you received?
   Bad _____ Poor _____ Fair _____ Good _____ Excellent ✓
10. How did you hear about us? John Richards
11. Any additional comments:

Patient's Initials: DM Tech Initials: JR

Thank you!!

2. Sleep Study Results Form

Revere Health
Let's live better.

Patient Name: David Meine
Date: November 28, 2017
Tech: Jessica Migliaccio

Time	Epoch	Stage	SaO2	HR	Resp	CPAP	Leak	EPR	Body	Events & Observations
10:09	1	Wake	93	65	8				Supine	Pt and machine calibrations done. Impedance check done. Lights off. Begin study.
10:29	41	N2	90	62	8				Supine	PT has fallen asleep. PT has had desats with what appear to be hypopneas. Pt has had moderate snoring. Pt has had some arousals.
10:49	81	N2	86	63	12				Supine	Pt has had desats with what appear to be hypopneas. Pt has had some central apneas. PT has had severe snoring. Pt has had arousals.
11:09	121	Wake	84	58	10				Supine	PT has had desats with what appear to be hypopneas, and central apneas. PT has had limb movements, and arousals. PT has had severe snoring.
11:29	161	N2	93	57	6				Supine	PT has had desats with what appear to be hypopneas, and central apneas. Pt has had limb movements, and arousals. Oxygen has been going into the 80s.
11:49	201	N2	87	61	12				Supine	PT has had moderate snoring. PT has had desats with what appear to be hypopneas. PT has had arousals. Oxygen has been going into the 80s.
12:09	241	N1	93	58	8	5.0	3	6	Supine	Tech in room to put pt on CPAP. Pt is wearing the Airfit F20 medium. Pt has had desats with what appear to be central apneas. Pt has had arousals.
12:29	281	N2	92	59	12	6.0	3	4	Supine	Tech raised pressure to 6.0 cm to see if it will help him stay asleep. Pt has had desats with what appear to be central apneas. PT has had arousals.
12:49	321	N2	91	63	12	7.0	3	6	Supine	Tech raised pressure to 7.0 cm for snoring. Pt has had some mild snoring. Oxygen has been in the 90s.
1:09	361	Wake	86	68	6	7.0	3	30	Supine	PT has had desats with what appear to be central apneas. Pt has moved around a little and his mask has started to leak a little. Tech in room to fix.
1:29	401	N1	86	58	6	7.0	3	5	Supine	PT has gone into what appears to be REM. PT has had arousals. TP has had desats with what appear to be central apneas.
1:49	441	REM	90	59	10	7.0	3	6	Supine	PT has had desats with what appear to be hypopneas. TP has had limb movements, and arousals.
2:09	481	N2	90	59	12	Epap min/max 5.0/9.0	PS min/max 0/15.0	5	Supine	Tech changed pt to ASV for central apneas. Pt has had some desats with what appear to be central apneas and hypopneas. PT has had arousals. Oxygen has been in the 90s.
2:29	521	N2	93	59	14	5.0/9.0	0/15.0	6	Left	PT has been moving from his back to the left side. PT has appeared to be doing well.

3. PULS Cardiac Test

PULS
CARDIAC TEST

Doctor **Steven Gundry MD**
has requested this report for
Meine, David
10/12/18 1027 PST

PATIENT INFORMATION		SPECIMEN INFORMATION		PRACTITIONER INFORMATION	
Name Meine, David		Collection Date/Time	10/08/18 1030 PST	Name	Gundry, Steven
Age 61	Sex M	Received Date/Time	10/09/18 1000 PST	Client ID	2224 International Heart & Lung
Fasting Status Y	DOB 12/10/1956	Report Date/Time	10/12/18 1027 PST	Address	555 E Tachevah Dr, 3 W103 Palm Springs, CA 92262
Accession ID 27588		Report Status	Final		

Patient Acute Coronary Syndrome (ACS) Profile is Elevated

PULS Score: 10.38%

Normal < 3.50%	Borderline 3.50% - 7.49%	Elevated ≥ 7.50%

Expected Score: 2.96%

TEST INTERPRETATION:

- Your PULS score indicates that **10.38%** (Absolute Risk) of individuals of your age, sex, and score had a cardiac event within a 5 year time period. Your expected score of **2.96%** is where you should be according to your current age and sex.
- Your PULS score indicates that you are **3.51** times (Relative Risk) more likely to experience an ACS (heart attack) than would be expected for your age and sex.
- This PULS score classifies you at **High** Risk by AHA/ACC Cardiovascular Risk Guidelines.

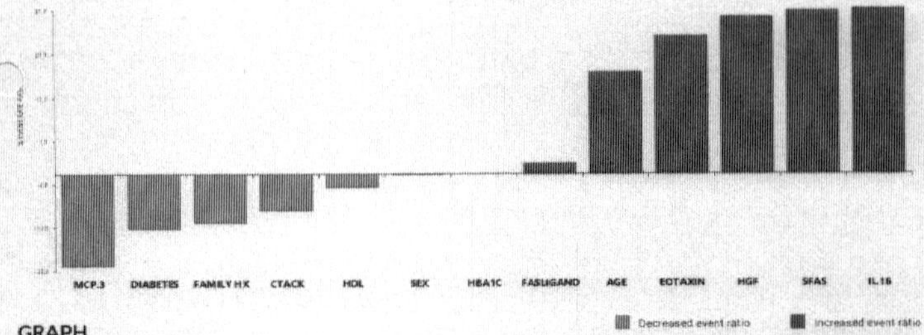

GRAPH

The size and location of each bar on the Protein Biomarker Graph indicates the relative impact of each biomarker in the formation & progression of cardiac lesions. The chart is read from right to left. Red bars above the zero line indicate factors that increase the probability of experiencing an Acute Coronary Syndrome (ACS). Green bars below the zero line indicate factors that decrease your probability of experiencing an ACS.

PULS CARDIAC TEST						PULS EXPECTED SCORE GAP		
PULS Score (Absolute Risk)	< 3.50%	3.50% - 7.49%	10.38 ≥ 7.50%	Expected Score For Age and Sex	2.96	Score Gap (Relative Risk)	3.51 < 5 Times	≥ 5 Times
AHA/ACC Guidelines Class	High	This patient is at high risk and should be treated as such. A low threshold for additional testing should be applied to this patient to better define the clinical picture and treatment plan. Aggressive lifestyle modification, supplements, and or medication should be considered. If the clinical situation warrants it, and the patient is not currently under the care of a cardiologist, referral to a cardiologist might be warranted.						

[illegible]

METHODOLOGY: Chemiluminescent Immunoassay and Photometry

[illegible]

Performing Laboratory: GD Biosciences, Inc. Irvine, CA - CLIA#05D2020794 - Lab Director: Douglas S. Harrington, M.D., FASPC, FCAP [illegible]

PULS
CARDIAC TEST

Doctor **Steven Gundry MD**
has requested this report for
Meine, David
10/12/18 1027 PST

PATIENT INFORMATION		SPECIMEN INFORMATION		PRACTITIONER INFORMATION	
Name Meine, David		Collection Date/Time	10/08/18 1030 PST	Name	Gundry, Steven
Age 61	Sex M	Received Date/Time	10/09/18 1000 PST	Client ID	2224 International Heart & Lung
Fasting Status Y	DOB 12/10/1956	Report Date/Time	10/12/18 1027 PST	Address	555 E Tachevah Dr. 3 W103 Palm Springs, CA 92262
Accession ID 27588		Report Status	Final		

ABOUT THIS TEST

The PULS Cardiac Score quantifies endothelial damage and predicts the likelihood of Acute Coronary Syndrome (ACS-heart attack, unstable angina & sudden cardiac death) within 5 years. The PULS Cardiac test measures the body's immune response pathway of coronary endothelial damage causing the formation, progression & likelihood of cardiac lesion rupture that can lead to a heart attack.

PROTEIN RESULTS		(RELATIVE % CONTRIBUTION TO THE PULS SCORE)		
PULS Biomarker	**Relation To Endothelial Damage & Unstable Cardiac Lesions**	**Normal**	**Borderline**	**Elevated**
MEASURES IMMUNE FORMATION & FREE RADICAL DAMAGE				
IL-16	Signaling molecule that triggers the repair process; often associated with stress, obesity, and sleep apnea			52.58
MEASURES IMMUNE RESPONSE				
MCP-3	Recruits monocyte/macrophages that form foam cells to clean up damaged cells, lipids, and cellular debris	21.20		
Eotaxin	Recruits eosinophils that consume fibrin and facilitates repair			31.71
CTACK	Recruits T-cells that regulate the local inflammatory response at the site of a lesion	8.47		
MEASURES DISEASE PROGRESSION				
Fas	Soluble form prevents programmed cell death (apoptosis) - usually indicates healing			37.71
FasLigand	Initiates programmed cell death and recycling - associated with more acute processes		2.48	
HGF	Governs tissue remodeling & repair			36.19
MEASURES INSULIN SENSITIVITY (%)				
HBA1c	Helps define insulin sensitivity and increased values indicate increased risk		6	
MEASURES METABOLIC RISK FACTOR (mg/dL)		LOW		NORMAL
HDL	Helps remove damaged cholesterol and neutralizes free radicals			50

TEST COMMENTS

[illegible]

METHODOLOGY: Chemiluminescent Immunoassay and Photometry

[illegible]

Performing Laboratory: GD Biosciences, Inc. Irvine, CA - CLIA#05D2020794 - Lab Director: Douglas S. Harrington, M.D., FASPC, FCAP

4. Salveo Diagnostics Report:

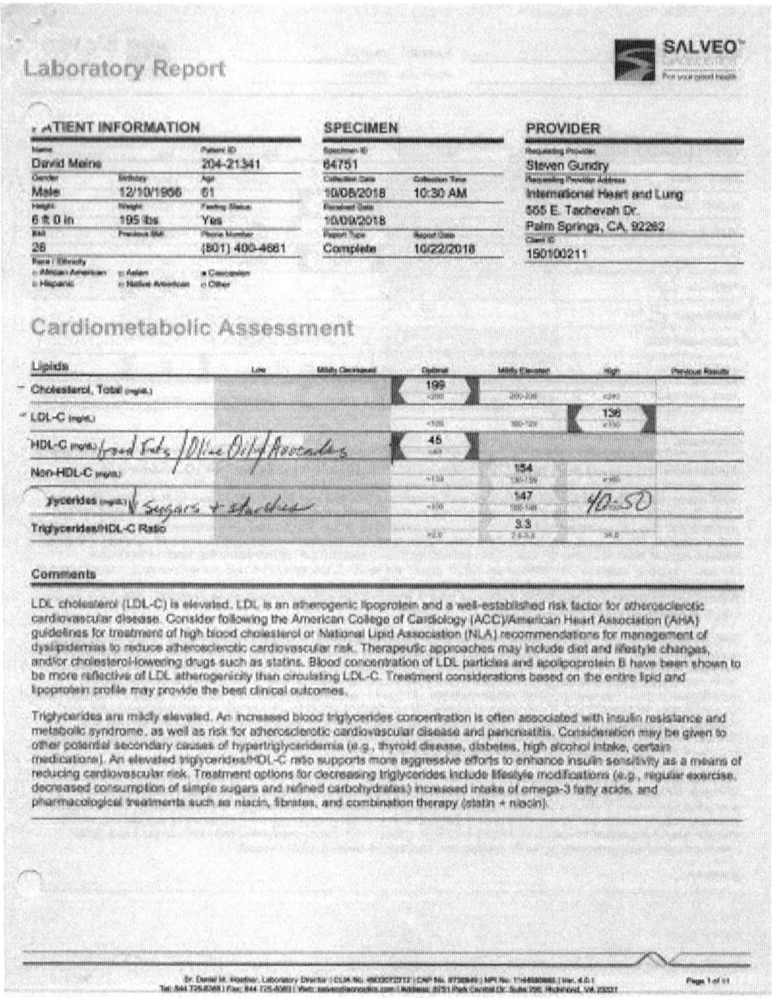

Laboratory Report

SALVEO™

PATIENT INFORMATION

Name		Patient ID
David Meine		204-21341
Gender	Birthday	Age
Male	12/10/1966	61
Height	Weight	Fasting Status
6 ft 0 in	195 lbs	Yes
BMI	Previous BMI	Phone Number
26		(801) 400-4661

Race / Ethnicity: ☐ African American ☐ Asian ■ Caucasian ☐ Hispanic ☐ Native American ☐ Other

SPECIMEN

Specimen ID	
64751	
Collection Date	Collection Time
10/08/2018	10:30 AM
Received Date	
10/09/2018	
Report Type	Report Date
Complete	10/22/2018

PROVIDER

Requesting Provider: Steven Gundry

Requesting Provider Address: International Heart and Lung, 555 E. Tachevah Dr., Palm Springs, CA, 92262

Client ID: 150100211

Cardiometabolic Assessment

Lipids	Low	Mildly Decreased	Optimal	Mildly Elevated	High	Previous Results
Cholesterol, Total (mg/dL)			199			
LDL-C (mg/dL)					136	
HDL-C (mg/dL) Good Fats / Olive Oil / Avocados			45			
Non-HDL-C (mg/dL)				154		
Triglycerides (mg/dL) ↓ Sugars + starches				147	40:50	
Triglycerides/HDL-C Ratio				3.3		

Comments

LDL cholesterol (LDL-C) is elevated. LDL is an atherogenic lipoprotein and a well-established risk factor for atherosclerotic cardiovascular disease. Consider following the American College of Cardiology (ACC)/American Heart Association (AHA) guidelines for treatment of high blood cholesterol or National Lipid Association (NLA) recommendations for management of dyslipidemias to reduce atherosclerotic cardiovascular risk. Therapeutic approaches may include diet and lifestyle changes, and/or cholesterol-lowering drugs such as statins. Blood concentration of LDL particles and apolipoprotein B have been shown to be more reflective of LDL atherogenicity than circulating LDL-C. Treatment considerations based on the entire lipid and lipoprotein profile may provide the best clinical outcomes.

Triglycerides are mildly elevated. An increased blood triglycerides concentration is often associated with insulin resistance and metabolic syndrome, as well as risk for atherosclerotic cardiovascular disease and pancreatitis. Consideration may be given to other potential secondary causes of hypertriglyceridemia (e.g., thyroid disease, diabetes, high alcohol intake, certain medications). An elevated triglycerides/HDL-C ratio supports more aggressive efforts to enhance insulin sensitivity as a means of reducing cardiovascular risk. Treatment options for decreasing triglycerides include lifestyle modifications (e.g., regular exercise, decreased consumption of simple sugars and refined carbohydrates) increased intake of omega-3 fatty acids, and pharmacological treatments such as niacin, fibrates, and combination therapy (statin + niacin).

Page 1 of 11

Name David Meine | Patient ID 204-21341

Specimen ID 64751 | Report Date 10/22/2018

SALVEO™ DIAGNOSTICS
For your good health

Other Lipoprotein Markers	Low	Mildly Decreased	Optimal	Mildly Elevated	High	Previous Results
LDL-P * (nmol/L)			<1100	1366 1100-1399	≥1400	
Lp(a)-P * (nmol/L)			<45 <50	50-80	>80	
VLDL-P * (nmol/L)			<150	221 150-299	≥300	
IDL-P * (nmol/L)			144 <150	150-299	≥300	
ApoB (mg/dL) LDL			≤59	60-79	94 ≥80	
ApoA-I (mg/dL) HDL	<114	124 114-131	>131			
ApoB/ApoA-I Ratio			≤0.60	0.76 0.61-0.80	>0.80	
sdLDL-C * (mg/dL) ↓ sugars / butter / cheese / Coconut Oil / MCT Oil			[illegible]	21-30	43 ≥31	
ApoE Genotype * No risk of Alzheimer's			3/3 3/3	2/2, 2/3, 2/4	3/4, 4/4	

Comments

Apolipoprotein B (apoB) and small, dense LDL cholesterol (sdLDL-C) concentrations are high, and LDL particles (LDL-P) are mildly elevated. ApoB concentration is often used as a surrogate marker of LDL-P as each LDL particle contains exactly one apoB protein, although it is important to note that apoB is also found in other atherogenic lipoproteins such as VLDL, IDL, and Lp(a). The sdLDL-C test measures the cholesterol in the small, potentially more atherogenic LDL particles. Many studies have demonstrated that each of these markers more accurately predict LDL atherogenicity and cardiovascular disease risk than does LDL cholesterol. LDL-P, apoB, and sdLDL-C are often higher in patients with insulin resistance, prediabetes, and type 2 diabetes mellitus, and are important goals of therapy. The National Lipid Association (NLA) recommends that apoB be used as a secondary target of treatment for dyslipidemia. LDL-P, apoB, and sdLDL-C concentrations may be decreased by regular exercise and reduced intake of refined carbohydrates and simple sugars. Pharmacological treatments include statins, niacin, ezetimibe, fibrates, and combination therapy (statin + niacin or statin + fibrate). Combination therapy may be particularly effective in lowering LDL-P and apoB, especially when small, dense LDL is present.

Very low-density lipoprotein particle concentration (VLDL-P) is mildly elevated. VLDL particles are triglyceride-rich lipoproteins that are synthesized by the liver and excreted into the bloodstream in response to bodily energy demands. VLDL particles have a half-life of approximately 6 hours and are metabolized to intermediate-density lipoprotein (IDL) particles (remnant lipoproteins) which are cleared from the blood by the liver or are converted to LDL particles. Elevated VLDL-P may result from familial hypertriglyceridemia or familial combined lipoproteinemia, or may be seen in patients with mild lipoprotein lipase or apolipoprotein CII deficiencies. Increased VLDL-P may also be triggered by conditions such as insulin resistance, metabolic syndrome, and diabetes, or by agents such as estrogens, glucocorticoids, excessive alcohol, or anabolic steroids. Lifestyle changes (e.g., increased exercise and Mediterranean diet, with reduced intake of refined carbohydrates), treatment of the underlying condition, or removal of a triggering agent may effectively reduce VLDL-P.

Apolipoprotein A-I (apoA-I) is mildly decreased. ApoA-I is the major protein component of HDL particles and may be used as a surrogate measure of HDL particle concentration. It is important for cholesterol transport and has potent anti-inflammatory properties. Low apoA-I levels are associated with insulin resistance, metabolic syndrome, and increased risk for cardiovascular events. Low apoA-I in the setting of normal HDL-C suggests that the HDL present may not be functioning in a cardioprotective manner. ApoA-I concentration may be increased by regular exercise and dietary supplementation with omega-3 fatty acids; pharmacological treatments include niacin, fibrates, and combination therapy (statin + niacin).

Continued...

Dr. Daniel M. Hoefner, Laboratory Director | CLIA No. 49D2072312 | CAP No. 8730849 | NPI No. 1144680885 | Ver. 4.0.1
Tel: 844.725-8365 | Fax: 844.725-8363 | Web: salveodiagnostics.com | Address: 8751 Park Central Dr. Suite 200, Richmond, VA 23227

Page 2 of 11

Name	David Meine	Patient ID	204-21341
Specimen ID	64751	Report Date	10/22/2018

SALVEO™ DIAGNOSTICS For your good health

Comments

C-reactive protein (CRP) and fibrinogen are mildly elevated. Although both markers are elevated in response to inflammation, and predict risk of cardiovascular disease and associated events, they have unique properties and functions. Both may be elevated by one inflammatory event, but each may be selectively elevated in response to different stimuli. This result is suggestive of increased inflammation and/or infection that may be accompanied by increased blood viscosity. Inflammatory bowel disease and related conditions have also been shown to increase serum levels of these markers. If abdominal symptoms are present, consider a Salveo Diagnostics™ Gut Health Assessment.

CRP is the most sensitive marker of systemic inflammation, yet it is non-specific and has a relatively short half-life of about 20 hours. Values may increase markedly (1000X or more) in response to any form of acute inflammation (e.g., infections, trauma, malignancy, smoking) and return to normal in as little as one week. In the setting of chronic inflammation (e.g., rheumatoid arthritis, obesity), CRP values tend to be mildly elevated and remain so for the duration of the inflammation. Thus, it has been recommended to check CRP level 2-4 weeks after the first elevated value to determine if the elevation is persistent, which would be consistent with chronic inflammation. High baseline hs-CRP values are a strong predictor of cardiovascular events and worsening disease progression in patients with insulin resistance, metabolic syndrome, and other chronic diseases.

Fibrinogen, an acute-phase protein produced in the liver and the building block of blood clots, increases in response to inflammation but is not as sensitive to inflammation as C-reactive protein (CRP). Fibrinogen has a longer half-life than CRP, and baseline blood concentrations that are much higher (2500-3500X) than those of CRP. This is because of fibrinogen's extremely important role in the coagulation process, which the body uses to protect itself from bleeding excessively after injury. In addition, because of its high molecular weight and butterfly-like structure, fibrinogen is one of the key factors influencing blood viscosity. Elevations in fibrinogen in response to inflammation can thus be very problematic, slowing blood flow and promoting the formation of abnormal clots in the coronary and other vasculature. In fact, elevated fibrinogen has consistently been shown to be a significant predictor of adverse cardiovascular conditions (e.g., hypertension) and events (e.g., deep-vein thrombosis, heart attack, and stroke).

Treatment should focus on decreasing inflammation. Lifestyle changes are often the most effective anti-inflammatory therapy, including regular and consistent exercise, weight reduction, smoking cessation, and an anti-inflammatory diet rich in fresh fruits and vegetables, vitamin C, omega-3 fatty acids, soluble fiber, nuts, and spices (e.g., Mediterranean diet). Statin therapy has been associated with decreased levels of CRP and fibrinogen, and may be appropriate depending on patient presentation and other laboratory values. Fibrates may be especially helpful in lowering serum fibrinogen levels.

Homocysteine is mildly elevated. Homocysteine is an amino acid byproduct of methionine metabolism and is normally recycled into methionine or converted to cysteine with the aid of B-vitamin cofactors. Elevated blood homocysteine level increases susceptibility to inflammation and oxidative stress that is associated with a variety of age-related conditions, including hypertension, renal disease, osteoporosis, cognitive decline, and dementia. Mild-to-moderate hyperhomocysteinemia may also stem from poor diet, hypothyroidism, certain drugs, or DNA variants of the methylenetetrahydrofolate reductase (*MTHFR*) gene. Chronic elevations of homocysteine may lead to endothelial dysfunction, vascular injury, and thrombogenicity, increasing risk for cardiovascular events and strokes. In addition to aggressive treatment of other cardiovascular risk factors, regular exercise, an anti-inflammatory diet, supplemental B vitamins (a B-vitamin complex, along with B_6 and methylated forms of folate, B_{12}, and/or betaine if *MTHFR* polymorphisms are present), and vitamin D may help prevent diseases of aging associated with elevated homocysteine.

Continued...

Dr. Daniel M. Hoefner, Laboratory Director | CLIA No. 49D2072312 | CAP No. 8730849 | NPI No. 1144680885 | Ver. 4.0.1
Tel: 844 725-8365 | Fax: 844 725-8363 | Web: salveodiagnostics.com | Address: 8751 Park Central Dr. Suite 200, Richmond, VA 23227

Name David Meine | Patient ID 204-21341
Specimen ID 64751 | Report Date 10/22/2018

SALVEO™ DIAGNOSTICS
For your good health

Comments

Continued...

This patient is homozygous (T/T) for the methylenetetrahydrofolate reductase *(MTHFR)* C677T polymorphism. The *MTHFR* gene encodes an enzyme that helps convert folic acid to its active form (L-methylfolate), important for methylation of DNA, RNA, and proteins, as well as the remethylation of homocysteine to methionine in the folate metabolic pathway. The C677T polymorphism reduces MTHFR activity, which can lead to decreased production of L-methylfolate and a build-up of homocysteine (especially in the homozygous state). L-methylfolate deficiency may also affect DNA synthesis/repair, antioxidant synthesis, and immune activity, increasing susceptibility to hypertension, certain cancers, and neural tube defects in the unborn child. It may also cause a reduced or adverse response to certain drugs. In addition, decreased methylation capability may impair production of neurotransmitters, increasing risk for disorders of mood and cognition (e.g., depression, dementia, memory/attention deficits). Patients who are homozygous for this *MTHFR* polymorphism are likely to have elevated homocysteine levels, especially if folate intake is inadequate. Such patients may not respond sufficiently to supplementation with folic acid and may receive greater benefit from the active L-methylfolate in combination with methylcobalamin (methylated B_{12}) and vitamin B_6, important cofactors in the folate metabolic pathway. Other homocysteine-lowering treatments include betaine and riboflavin, which has been shown to reduce high blood pressure in 677 T/T homozygotes.

Diabetes / Insulin Resistance	Low	Mildly Decreased	Optimal	Mildly Elevated	High	Previous Results
Glucose (mg/dL)	≤60	61-70	71-99	115 100-125	≥126	
HbA1c (%) 2 months of sugars + proteins before the test				5.9 5.7-6.4	5.0↓	
Insulin (µU/mL)	<1	1-3	4-9	10 10-11	≥12	
Fructosamine (µmol/L) 2 weeks of sugars			≤265	292 266-307	≥308	
HOMA-IR			<2.5	2.8 2.5-3.9	≥4.0	
C-Peptide (ng/mL)	<1		2.31 1.00-2.69	2.70-2.99	≥3.00	
Adiponectin * (µg/mL)	≤5	8 6-8	9-49		≥50	
Leptin * (ng/mL)			5 <15	15-35	≥36	
IGF-1 (ng/mL)	<63		191 63-245		>245	
Free Fatty Acids (µmol/L)			≤0.55	0.58 0.56-0.71	≥0.72	
Proinsulin * (pmol/L)			≤13	20 14-20	≥21	
Proinsulin/C-Peptide Ratio			<3.6	3.6-4.9	~~8.5~~	
Anti-GAD Antibody (IU/mL)			<5 ≤5		>5	

Dr. Daniel M. Hoefner, Laboratory Director | CLIA No. 49D2072312 | CAP No. 8730849 | NPI No. 1144680885 | Ver. 4.0.1
Tel: 844 725-8365 | Fax: 844 725-8363 | Web: salveodiagnostics.com | Address: 8751 Park Central Dr. Suite 200, Richmond, VA 23227

Page 5 of 11

Name	David Meine	Patient ID	204-21341
Specimen ID	64751	Report Date	10/22/2018

SALVEO™

For your good health

Comments

The glucose, hemoglobin A1c (HbA1c), and fructosamine (glycated serum proteins) concentrations are elevated, consistent with the American Diabetes Association (ADA) criteria for prediabetes. Chronic hyperglycemia has been associated with premature aging and increased risk for cardiovascular disease. Fructosamine level is a useful indicator of treatment response in the short-term, as it has been shown to be a sensitive marker of glycemic control over the course of a 2- to 3- week period (including large glucose excursions). Consider ADA guidelines for achieving appropriate glycemic control.

Insulin concentration is mildly elevated. Fasting insulin in this range may be an early indicator of insulin resistance and risk for progression to type 2 diabetes. The Homeostatic Model Assessment of Insulin Resistance (HOMA-IR) is also mildly increased, consistent with insulin resistance. HOMA-IR uses fasting glucose and insulin measures to estimate whole body insulin resistance by modeling the balance between hepatic glucose output, insulin secretion, and glucose uptake in peripheral tissue. These values should be viewed in the context of the patient's clinical presentation and other biomarker values (e.g., leptin, adiponectin, lipoprotein particles).

Proinsulin concentration is mildly elevated, and the proinsulin/C-peptide ratio is high. Proinsulin is the precursor to insulin—synthesized in pancreatic beta cells, packaged into secretory granules, and proteolytically cleaved into insulin (and C-peptide) over the course of many hours. Typically, levels of circulating proinsulin tend to be a small fraction of insulin levels. Serum proinsulin rises with age and is a highly sensitive and early indicator of beta-cell dysfunction and insulin resistance. An increase in the proinsulin/C-peptide ratio reflects reduced efficiency of proinsulin-to-insulin processing inside the pancreatic beta cells and/or dysregulated secretory mechanisms leading to release of immature secretory granules. Elevated proinsulin and proinsulin/C-peptide ratios are both risk factors for development of type 2 diabetes and, in patients with prediabetes or diabetes, for incident coronary heart disease. Hyperproinsulinemia may also be seen in patients with pancreatic tumors, chronic renal failure, cirrhosis of the liver, or hyperthyroidism. Consider approaches to reduce glycemic load and improve insulin sensitivity (i.e., reduced dietary intake of simple/refined carbohydrates, increased exercise, and perhaps pharmacologic therapies) to reduce beta-cell strain.

Adiponectin is mildly decreased. Adiponectin is an anti-inflammatory adipokine secreted by adipose tissue that protects endothelial function, inhibits atherogenesis, and enhances insulin sensitivity. Metabolically unfavorable conditions can lead to a decrease in adiponectin secretion. Low levels of adiponectin may contribute to type 2 diabetes and can precede other markers of insulin resistance. Lifestyle modification, visceral fat reduction, and certain medications can increase serum adiponectin and improve insulin sensitivity, thus helping to prevent both type 2 diabetes and cardiovascular disease.

Non-esterified "free" fatty acid concentration is mildly elevated. Free fatty acids are an important energy source for many tissues. Plasma free fatty acid levels are dynamically regulated by a number of factors including release from adipose tissue, lipolysis of lipoprotein-associated triglycerides, and recent dietary fat intake. Elevated free fatty acids in the fasting state have been associated with the metabolic syndrome and can promote insulin resistance, inflammation, and increased risk for diabetes.

Cardiac Stress	Low	Mildly Decreased	Optimal	Mildly Elevated	High	Previous Results
NT-proBNP (pg/mL)			<5 [illegible]	[illegible]	[illegible]	

Page 6 of 11

Name: David Minkoff Patient ID: 204-21341

Specimen ID: 84751 Report Date: 10/22/2018

SALVEO DIAGNOSTICS

For your good health

RBC Fatty Acid Profile

RBC Fatty Acid Profile	Low	Mildly Decreased	Optimal	Mildly Elevated	High	Previous Results
RBC Omega-3 Index (%)	[illegible]	7.6 [illegible]	[illegible]	10-12		
Omega-3 Total (%)	[illegible]		10.70 [illegible]		[illegible]	
Alpha Linolenic (ALA) (%)	[illegible]		0.20 [illegible]		[illegible]	
Eicosapentaenoic (EPA) (%)	[illegible]		1.30 [illegible]		[illegible]	
Docosapentaenoic (DPA) (%)	[illegible]		2.90 [illegible]		[illegible]	
Docosahexaenoic (DHA) (%)	[illegible]		6.30 [illegible]		[illegible]	
Omega-6 Total (%)	[illegible]		31.30 [illegible]		[illegible]	
Arachidonic (AA) (%)	[illegible]		13.50 [illegible]		[illegible]	
Linoleic (LA) (%)	[illegible]		13.60 [illegible]		[illegible]	
Cis-Monounsaturated Total (%)	[illegible]		15.20 [illegible]		[illegible]	
Saturated Total (%)	[illegible]		42.20 [illegible]		[illegible]	
D5 Desaturase Ratio (D5D)	[illegible]	[illegible]	9.00 [illegible]			
Desaturase Ratio (D6D)			0.000 [illegible]	[illegible]	[illegible]	

Comments

The omega-3 index (an indicator of average circulating omega-3 fatty acid levels over the past 2-3 months) is mildly decreased. Omega-3 fatty acids are important constituents of cell membranes in the body, where the correct fatty acid composition is vital to cardiometabolic and overall health. Low omega-3 fatty acid levels have been associated in many studies with increased risk for heart disease, stroke, sudden cardiac death, dementia, and even reduced life span. The omega-3 index is an accurate biomarker of omega-3 fatty acid intake and a cardiovascular risk marker that can be used as a target of therapy. Omega-3 fatty acid status can be improved by increasing consumption of "oily" fish (e.g., salmon, herring, tuna, mackerel), certain vegetable oils (e.g., olive and walnut), or with dietary supplements.

Lab Notes

The RBC Fatty Acid Profile was determined by OmegaQuant, LLC, 5009 W 12th Street, Sioux Falls, SD 57106, CLIA# 43D1106229. Reference ranges for components (other than the Omega-3 Index and desaturase ratios) were determined in a large clinical cohort (Harris et al., 2013. Prostaglandins Leukot Essent Fatty Acids; 88:257-263).

Hemostasis and Thrombosis

Hemostasis and Thrombosis	Low	Mildly Decreased	Optimal	Mildly Elevated	High	Previous Results
Factor V Leiden *			Arg/Arg [illegible]		[illegible]	
Factor II (Prothrombin) *			G/G [illegible]		[illegible]	

Page 7 of 11

Name	David Meine	Patient ID	204-21341
Specimen ID	64751	Report Date	10/22/2018

SALVEO™ For your good health

Cholesterol Homeostasis	Low	Mildly Decreased	Optimal	Mildly Elevated	High	Previous Results
Sitosterol * (ug/mL)	[illegible]		2.77 [illegible]		[illegible]	
Campesterol * (ug/mL)	[illegible]		3.88 [illegible]		[illegible]	
Cholestanol * (ug/mL)	[illegible]		2.50 [illegible]		[illegible]	
Desmosterol (ug/mL)	[illegible]		[illegible]		2.12 [illegible]	

Comments

Concentration of desmosterol is elevated, indicating cholesterol hypersynthesis. Serum cholesterol may be obtained through the diet (by absorption) or may be synthesized by the cells of the body. An individual's genetic makeup influences whether serum cholesterol concentration is derived predominately through absorption or synthesis. To properly treat serum cholesterol elevations, it is important to know the major source of the cholesterol (synthesis, absorption, or both). Desmosterol is an intermediate molecule in the synthetic pathway of cholesterol and can thus serve as a surrogate marker of cholesterol synthesis. Patients who are "cholesterol hypersynthesizers" are likely to benefit from the use of statins, which inhibit cholesterol synthesis, as a lipid-lowering therapy. Note that statin monotherapy may induce compensatory cholesterol hyperabsorption, thus follow-up sterol testing may be advised to monitor treatment.

Gut Health Serum Assessment

Celiac Disease	Low	Mildly Decreased	Optimal	Mildly Elevated	High	Previous Results
Anti-tTG (IgG) (U)			5 [illegible]	[illegible]	[illegible]	
Anti-tTG (IgA) (U)			[illegible]	25 [illegible]	[illegible]	
Anti-DGP (IgG) (U)			6 [illegible]	[illegible]	[illegible]	
Anti-DGP (IgA) (U)			16 [illegible]	[illegible]	[illegible]	

Comments

There is some serological evidence for the presence of gluten-sensitive enteropathy (celiac disease). The use of anti-DGP in combination with anti-tTG increases diagnostic accuracy and may rule out the need for biopsy in more than 92% of individuals. Isolated anti-tTG has also been described to occur infrequently in conditions such as other autoimmune disorders, infections, etc. The ACG guidelines suggest that diagnostic testing for celiac disease should be performed with patients on a gluten-containing diet; but, for monitoring purposes, patients are expected to adhere to a gluten-free diet.

Autoimmune Assessment

Rheumatoid Arthritis	Low	Mildly Decreased	Optimal	Mildly Elevated	High	Previous Results
Anti-CCP (3.1) (U)			11 [illegible]	[illegible]	[illegible]	
Rheumatoid Factor (IU/mL)			<10 [illegible]		[illegible]	

[illegible] Page 8 of 11

Name	David Meine	Patient ID	204-21341
Specimen ID	64751	Report Date	10/22/2018

SALVEO DIAGNOSTICS
For your good health

Thyroid Health Assessment

Thyroid Workup	Low	Mildly Decreased	Optimal	Mildly Elevated	High	Previous Results
TSH (µIU/mL)	≤0.400	0.401-0.600	1.410 0.601-2.499	2.500-3.999	≥4.000	
T4, Total (µg/dL)	≤4.9		8.0 5.0-11.6		≥11.7	
T4, Free (ng/dL)	<0.93		0.97 0.93-1.70		>1.70	
T3, Total (ng/dL)	≤77		145 78-179		≥180	
T3, Free (pg/mL)	≤2.0		3.2 2.1-4.3		≥4.4	

Hormonal Health Assessment

	Low	Mildly Decreased	Optimal	Mildly Elevated	High	Previous Results
PSA, Total (ng/mL)			0.9 ≤2.6	2.7-4.0	≥4.1	
Testosterone, Total (ng/dL)	<350		684 350-1200		>1200	
Testosterone, Free (ng/dL)	<4.70		9.59 4.70-24.40		>24.40	
SHBG (nmol/L)	≤17		64 18-130		≥131	
DHEA * (ng/dL)			106 <650		≥650	
DHEA-S (µg/dL)	≤44		121 45-456		≥457	
Pregnenolone * (ng/dL)	<48		48 48-330		>330	
Estradiol (pg/mL) Ginkgo Biloba 120mg 2 a day		<30	40.5 <50		≥50	
LH (IU/L)	≤1.7		8.0 1.7-8.6		>8.6	
Prolactin (ng/mL)	<4.00		6.73 4.00-15.20		>15.20	
Progesterone (ng/mL)	<0.09		0.34 0.09-1.49		>1.49	

Bone Health Assessment

Bone Health	Low	Mildly Decreased	Optimal	Mildly Elevated	High	Previous Results
PTH, Intact (pg/mL)	≤15		35 15-64		≥65	

Dr. Daniel M. Hoefner, Laboratory Director | CLIA No. 49D2072312 | CAP No. 8736849 | NPI No. 1144880685 | Ver. 4.0.1
Tel: 844 725-8365 | Fax: 844 725-8363 | Web: salveodiagnostics.com | Address: 8751 Park Central Dr. Suite 200, Richmond, VA 23227

Page 9 of 11

Name	David Meine	Patient ID	204-21341
Specimen ID	64751	Report Date	10/22/2018

SALVEO™ DIAGNOSTICS
For your good health

Metabolic Profiles

Electrolytes	Low	Mildly Decreased	Optimal	Mildly Elevated	High	Previous Results
Sodium (Na+) (mmol/L)	≤136		140 137-144		≥145	
Phosphorus (mg/dL)	≤2.4	2.5-2.8	3.0 2.9-4.1	4.2-4.5	≥4.6	
Potassium (K+) (mmol/L)	≤3.5		4.1 3.6-5.0		≥5.1	
Bicarbonate (HCO3-) (mmol/L)	≤21		27 22-30		≥31	
Chloride (Cl-) (mmol/L)	≤98		105 99-106		≥107	
Anion Gap (Calculation) (mmol/L)	≤5.0		8.0 5.1-18.9		≥19.0	
Calcium (Ca2+) (mg/dL)	6.5-8.6	8.7-8.9	9.5 9.0-9.9	10.0-10.2	10.3-13.0	
Magnesium (Mg2+) (mg/dL)	≤1.90	1.91-2.04	2.44 2.05-2.55	2.56-2.69	≥2.70	

Kidney Function	Low	Mildly Decreased	Optimal	Mildly Elevated	High	Previous Results
Blood Urea Nitrogen (BUN) (mg/dL)	≤7		22 8-24		≥25	
Creatinine (mg/dL)			1.18 <1.31		≥1.31	
BUN/Creatinine Ratio	≤10.0		18.6 10.1-33.2		≥33.3	
Cystatin C (mg/L)			0.90 ≤0.95	0.96-1.03	>1.03	
eGFR (based on Cystatin C) (mL per minute per1.73 m^2)	≤60	86 61-90	≥91			

Good marker

Comments

The mildly decreased value for estimated GFR is based on the CKD-EPI-Cys calculation that is normalized to an average body surface area (BSA) of 1.73 m^2.

Liver Assessment	Low	Mildly Decreased	Optimal	Mildly Elevated	High	Previous Results
ALT (U/L)			19 <30	30-49	≥50	
AST (U/L)			20 <40		≥40	
ALP (U/L)		≤28	85 29-98		≥99	
GGT (U/L)			10.0 <51	51-60	≥61	
Bilirubin, Total (mg/dL)			0.4 <1.3		≥1.3	
AST/ALT Ratio	≤0.7	0.8-0.9	1.1 1.0-1.9		≥2	

Name	David Meine	Patient ID	204-21341
Specimen ID	64751	Report Date	10/22/2018

SALVEO™ DIAGNOSTICS
For your good health

Proteins	Low	Mildly Decreased	Optimal	Mildly Elevated	High	Previous Results
Total Protein (g/dL)	≤5.9		6.0-7.7		7.8 (≥7.8)	
Albumin (g/dL)	≤3.6		4.6 (3.7-4.9)		≥5.0	
Globulin (g/dL)	≤1.7		3.2 (1.8-3.3)		≥3.4	
A/G Ratio	≤1.22		1.44 (1.23 - 2.41)		≥2.42	

Comments

Total protein is elevated, though neither albumin nor globulin (the non-albumin proteins such as immunoglobulins, carrier proteins, and acute phase reactants) exceed their respective reference intervals. Mild increases in albumin are most commonly a sign of dehydration, while globulin increases may indicate poor digestion/absorption (e.g., impaired protein digestion due to hypochlorhydria), liver dysfunction (increased immunoglobulin production in response to cellular damage), or increased oxidative stress.

Iron Studies	Low	Mildly Decreased	Optimal	Mildly Elevated	High	Previous Results
Iron (µg/dL)	≤59		69 (60-157)		≥158	
rritin (ng/mL)	<18		36 (18-243)		>243	
TIBC (µg/dL)	≤250		251-449		453 (≥450)	
Transferrin (mg/dL)	≤203		287 (204-381)		≥382	

Comments

The total iron binding capacity (TIBC) is elevated, while transferrin concentration is optimal. Although transferrin is the primary vehicle for circulating iron, it is not an exact measure of TIBC because not all of the iron is bound by transferrin.

Complete Blood Count

Complete Blood Count	Low	Mildly Decreased	Optimal	Mildly Elevated	High	Previous Results
Hematocrit (%) No Anemia	≤38.4	38.5-39.9	49.3 (40.0-51.9)		≥52.0	

* This test was developed and its performance characteristics were determined by Salveo Diagnostics, Inc. The U.S. Food & Drug Administration (FDA) has determined that it is unnecessary to clear or approve this test. It is to be used for clinical purposes and should not be regarded as investigational or for research. Salveo Diagnostics, Inc. is certified under CLIA '88 to perform high complexity clinical laboratory testing (CLIA # 49D2072312).

Dr. Daniel M. Hoefner, Laboratory Director | CLIA No. 49D2072312 | CAP No. 8730849 | NPI No. 1144680885 | Ver. 4.0.1
Tel: 844 725-8365 | Fax: 844 725-8363 | Web: salveodiagnostics.com | Address: 8751 Park Central Dr, Suite 200, Richmond, VA 23227

Page 11 of 11

5. Veridia Diagnostics Report:

Veridia Diagnostics

FINAL REPORT DATE	10/13/2018 10:17	COLLECTED	10/08/2018 10:30
LAST REPRINT	10/13/2018 11:54	RECEIVED	10/09/2018 10:07
REPORT STATUS	Final	ACCESSION ID	1810090086

PATIENT
MEINE, DAVID A
2579 N TURNBERRY CT
LEHI, UT 84043
(801)400-4661

PATIENT ID: A614256

GENDER	DATE OF BIRTH	AGE
Male	12/10/1956	61

HEIGHT: 6 ft 0 in
WEIGHT: 195 lbs
BMI: 26
HOURS SINCE LAST ATE: 10

PHYSICIAN
THE INTERNATIONAL HEART AND LUNG INSTITUTE -
GUNDRY, STEVEN , MD
555 TACHEVAH DR 3W-103
PALM SPRINGS, CA 92262

CLIENT NUMBER	PHONE	FAX
1010	760-323-5553	760-323-5554

Results

BIOMARKER Units of Measure	PAST RESULTS	MOST RECENT RESULT 10/08/2018	REFERENCE RANGE	DIAGNOSTIC SPECTRUM	
Cardiac Function *Heart.*					
SMC Cardiac Troponin-I* pg/mL		0.8	0.0-3.7	0.8	Goal: <3.8
Inflammation *on the inside of blood vessels*					
SMC Endothelin* pg/mL		1.5	0.0-3.7	1.5	Goal: <3.8
SMC Interleukin-6* pg/mL		0.5	0.0-4.5	0.5	Goal: <4.6
SMC Interleukin-17A* pg/mL		0.3	0.0-1.9	0.3	Goal: <2.0
SMC Interleukin-10* pg/mL		0.58	0.27-2.80	0.58	
SMC TNF-alpha* pg/mL		1.1	0.0-2.9	1.1	Goal: <3.0

Flagging: (H) High (L) Low (C) Early Notification Normal Borderline Abnormal

Veridia Diagnostics, 106 East Old Settlers Blvd, D-106, Round Rock, TX 78664 Phone: 800-400-4344 Fax: 510-225-2948

* This test was developed and performance characteristics were determined by Veridia and is not FDA approved/cleared. The laboratory is regulated under CLIA as qualified to perform high-complexity testing. This test is used for clinical purposes and should not be regarded as investigational or for research. Results are not for use as the sole means for clinical diagnosis or patient management.

Laboratory Director: Mark Stene, Ph.D., Zach Liu, M.D. (NJ), CLIA: 05D2050618 CAP: 7229934 1

6. True Health Diagnostics

TRUE HEALTH™ DIAGNOSTICS

Laboratory Results

Patient			
Name: DAVID MEINE	Phone #:	Patient ID #: 18-282-0218	
Fasting Status: 14 HOURS	Gender: MALE	Birthdate: 12/10/1956	Age: 61
Height: 6 ft	Weight: 195 lbs	BMI: 26.4	Prev. BMI:

Specimen	
Collection Time: 10:30 am	Specimen ID: 18100900610
Collection Date: 10/8/2018	Report Type: COMPLETE
Received Date: 10/9/2018	Report Date: 10/11/2018

Provider
Requesting Provider: STEVEN GUNDRY, MD INTERNATIONAL HEART LUNG INSTITUTE 555 TACHEVAH DRIVE, 3W-103 PALM SPRINGS, CA 92262
Client ID: 06-92262-18-0006999

	Laboratory Test	Notes	High Risk	Intermediate Risk	Optimal	High Risk Range	Intermediate Risk Range	Optimal Range	Previous Results
Endothelial Function	Asymmetric Dimethylarginine (ng/mL)[rv]				90	> 108	97 - 108	< 97	
	Symmetric Dimethylarginine (ng/mL)[rv]			102		> 104	88 - 104	< 68	
	L-arginine (ng/mL)[rv]				11355	< 4500 or > 22500		4500 - 22500	
	Asymmetric Dimethylarginine/Arginine Ratio (calculated)[v]			~~7.9~~		> 9.8	7.8 - 9.8	< 7.8	
Myocardial Structure/Stress/Function	Galectin-3 (ng/mL)[v]	Good Gut Bugs			11.1	> 25.9	17.9 - 25.9	< 17.9	

Vital Reds / Olive Oil / Dark Chocolate / Red Wine / Black Coffee

Primal Plants + Prebiothrive

Lab Notes:

Provider Notes:

www.truehealthdiag.com

1 / 3

True Health Diagnostics LLC | Bobbie C. Sutton, MD, PhD | Laboratory Director | CLIA No. 45D2082195

© 2018 | 3803 Parkwood Blvd, Suite 400 | Frisco, TX 75034 | Phone: 1-877-443-5227 | Fax: 804-343-2704

TRUE HEALTH™ DIAGNOSTICS

Omega 3 and Omega 6 Fatty Acids Profile

Patient			
Name: DAVID MEINE	Phone #:	Patient ID #: 18-282-0218	
Fasting Status: 14 HOURS	Gender: MALE	Birthdate: 12/10/1956	Age: 61
Height: 6 ft	Weight: 195 lbs	BMI: 26.4	Prev. BMI:

Specimen	
Collection Time: 10:30 am	Specimen ID: 18100900610
Collection Date: 10/8/2018	Report Type: COMPLETE
Received Date: 10/9/2018	Report Date: 10/11/2018

Provider
Requesting Provider: STEVEN GUNDRY, MD
INTERNATIONAL HEART LUNG INSTITUTE
555 TACHEVAH DRIVE, 3W-103
PALM SPRINGS, CA 92262
Client ID: 06-92262-18-0006999

	Laboratory Test	Notes	High Risk	Intermediate Risk	Optimal	High Risk Range	Intermediate Risk Range	Optimal Range	Previous Results
Index	HS-Omega-3 Index[a,iv] (RBC EPA+DHA)[a]	Fish Oil		7.5		< 4.0%	4.0% - 8.0%	> 8.0%	

Comments:

Your HS-Omega-3 Index is below the target range of 8%.

The HS-Omega-3 Index is the EPA+DHA content of RBC membranes. Increasing the intake of EPA+DHA by 1/2 to 1 gram (500 - 1,000 mg) per day, from either oily fish or fish oil supplements, should significantly improve the index. The exact amount of EPA+DHA needed will vary person to person. A re-check should be done in 3 - 4 months.

Omega-3 Fatty Acids			
Fatty Acids	Range	Current	Previous
Omega-3 Total[v]	0.1% - 14.1%	**10.5%**	
Alpha-Linolenic (ALA)[iv]	0.1% - 0.4%	0.1%	
Docosapentaenoic (DPA)[iv]	0.6% - 4.1%	2.8%	
Eicosapentaenoic (EPA)[iv]	0.1% - 2.5%	1.4%	
Docosahexaenoic (DHA)[iv]	0.1% - 8.4%	6.1%	

Omega-6 Fatty Acids			
Fatty Acids	Range	Current	Previous
Omega-6 Total[v]	28.6% - 44.5%	**31.0%**	
Arachidonic (AA)[iv]	10.5% - 23.3%	13.4%	
Linoleic (LA)[iv]	4.6% - 21.3%	13.5%	

Other Fatty Acids			
Fatty Acids	Range	Current	Previous
cis-Monounsaturated Total[v]	11.5% - 20.5%	**15.8%**	
Saturated Total[v]	36.6% - 42.0%	**42.0%**	
Trans Total[v]	<0.1% - 1.8%	**0.7%**	

Content of EPA and DHA (mg/3 oz serving) in Fish[1]

Higher Omega-3	EPA	DHA	EPA+DHA
Herring, Pacific	1056	751	1807
Anchovy (canned in oil, European, drained solids)	649	1099	1748
Herring, Atlantic	773	939	1712
Salmon, Atlantic[2]	468	1227	1695
Salmon, Coho[2]	462	903	1365
Tuna, Bluefin	309	970	1279
Herring, Atlantic (pickled)	717	464	1181
Mackerel (canned, drained solids)	369	677	1046
Salmon, Sockeye	353	690	1043
Salmon, Chum (canned)	402	597	999
Salmon, Pink (canned, total can contents)	275	569	844
Sardines (canned in oil, Atlantic, drained solids w/bone)	402	433	835

Intermediate Omega-3	EPA	DHA	EPA+DHA
Swordfish[3]	108	656	764
Rainbow Trout (farmed)[4]	220	524	744
Tuna, White (canned in water, w/out salt)[3]	198	535	733
Sea Bass	175	473	648
Pollock, Atlantic	77	383	460
Oysters (farmed, eastern)[4]	195	179	374
Crab, King (cooked, moist heat)	251	100	351
Walleye	94	245	339
Crab, Dungeness (cooked, moist heat)	239	96	335
Flat Fish (flounder/sole)	143	112	255
Clams (cooked, moist heat)	117	124	241
Shrimp (mixed, cooked, moist heat)	115	120	235
Tuna, Light (canned, w/out salt)	40	190	230

Lower Omega-3	EPA	DHA	EPA+DHA
Halibut, Atlantic and Pacific	68	132	200
Northern Lobster (cooked, moist heat)	99	66	165
Scallops (cooked, steamed)	61	88	149
Catfish[4]	51	88	139
Haddock	43	93	136
Cod, Pacific	36	100	136
Cod, Atlantic	3	131	134
Mahi-Mahi (dolphin fish)	22	96	118
Tilapia	4	110	114
Orange Roughy	5	21	26

[1]From the USDA Nutrient Database. Values are for fish cooked with dry heat unless otherwise noted.
[2]This value averages EPA+DHA from farmed and wild fish.
[3]Because of the possibility for mercury contamination, the FDA and Environmental Protection Agency recommend that these fish (along with king mackerel and tilefish) not be consumed by women who are already or are trying to become pregnant, nursing mothers, and children under the age of two. For all other people, the intake of these fish should be limited to 6 oz. per week (or 12 oz. per week for albacore tuna).
[4]Although there has been some concern regarding the presence of small amounts of environmental pollutants in some types of farmed fish, the overall health benefit from the omega-3 fatty acids present in these fish has been calculated to far outweigh the risks (JAMA, 2006;296:1885-1899).

[a]The HS-Omega-3 Index cutpoints are based on Harris and von Shacky, Preventive Medicine 2004;39:212-220.

2 / 3

True Health Diagnostics LLC | Bobbie C. Sutton, MD, PhD | Laboratory Director | CLIA No. 45D2082195

7. Supplements Page

Supplements

Name: *David* Date: *12/5/18*

	Acetyl-L-Carnitine 250-500 mg/day
	Alpha Lipoic Acid (sustained release if you can find it) 300 mg/day
	Baby Aspirin once/day
	Biotin 5000 mg/day
	Borage oil 2,000 mg/ am & pm
	Curcumin
	Cholest-off two tablets twice/day (absorbs/blocks cholesterol) (at Costco)
	Chromium Picolinate 200-400 mcg/day
X	Cinnamon ¼ to ½ tsp/day – Cinsulin 1 twice a day (at Costco)
	Co-enzyme Q-10 100 mg/day
	DHEA 25 mg
X	Fish oil DHA 1,000 mg/day
	Flax Seed Oil 1,000 mg/day
	5-HTP
X	Ginkgo Biloba *120 mg 2 a day*
	Grape seed Extract 100 mg/day
	Green Tea Extract 200-500 mg/day
	Hawthorne 250-500 mg/day (Dr.'s Best/Clarks)
	Huperzine A 100 mcg/day
	Kaolic Garlic Heart Formula 106 two twice/day
	L-Reuteri (5 billion)
	Magnesium (potassium asporatate) 400 mg/day
X	Methyl B12 5,000 mcg Kirkland (Costco) sublingual *1 under tongue a day*
X	Methylfolate 1,000 mcg/day *1 a day*
	Milk Thistle
	Modified Citrus Pectin
	N-Acetyl-Cysteine (better known as NAC) 250-500 mg/day
	Niacin 500 mg
	No Flush Niacin 500 mg (extended release)
	Slo-Niacin 500 mg at night with 325 mg Tylenol *After two weeks increase to 1,000 mg
	Pregnenolone 50/100 mg
	Pycnogenol 25-50 mg/day
	Quercetin 500 mg 2/day
	Red Yeast Rice Extract 600 to 1,200 mg/day
	Relora
	Rhodiola 100-500 mg/day
	Selenium 200 mcg/day
	Spirulina
X	Tumeric Extract (curcumin) (With BioPerine) ~~900mg twice/day (Vitacost.com)~~ *You Theory @ Costco 3 a day*
X	Vit-C 1000 mg twice/day
	Vit-D3 5,000 IU, [illegible]/day *10,000 IUs daily*
	Vit-K2
	Schiff Digestive Advantage (Probiotic)
X	*Pau D'Arco 500mg 2 a day* → [illegible]
X	*Brassica Tea 2 cups daily (baltcoffee.com)*
X	*Vital Reds, Total Restore, Primal Plants, Lectin Shield*

6 months

8. PULS Report #2:

PULS CARDIAC TEST

Doctor **Steven Gundry MD**
has requested this report for
Meine, David
12/06/19 1235 PST

PATIENT INFORMATION		SPECIMEN INFORMATION		PRACTITIONER INFORMATION	
Name	Meine, David	Collection Date/Time	12/03/19 1323 PST	Name	Gundry, Steven
Age 62	Sex M	Received Date/Time	12/04/19 1000 PST	Client ID	2224 International Heart & Lung
DOB	12/10/1956	Report Date/Time	12/06/19 1235 PST	Address	555 E Tachevah Dr, 3 W103 Palm Springs, CA 92262
Accession ID	67881	Report Status	Final		

Patient Acute Coronary Syndrome (ACS) Profile is Elevated

PULS Score: 15.88%

Normal < 3.50%	Borderline 3.50% - 7.49%	Elevated ≥ 7.50%

Expected Score: 3.11%

TEST INTERPRETATION:

- Your PULS score indicates that **15.88%** (Absolute Risk) of individuals of your age, sex, and score had a cardiac event within a 5 year time period. Your expected score of **3.11%** is where you should be according to your current age and sex.
- Your PULS score indicates that you are **5.11** times (Relative Risk) more likely to experience an ACS (heart attack) than would be expected for your age and sex.
- This PULS score classifies you at **High** Risk by AHA/ACC Cardiovascular Risk Guidelines.

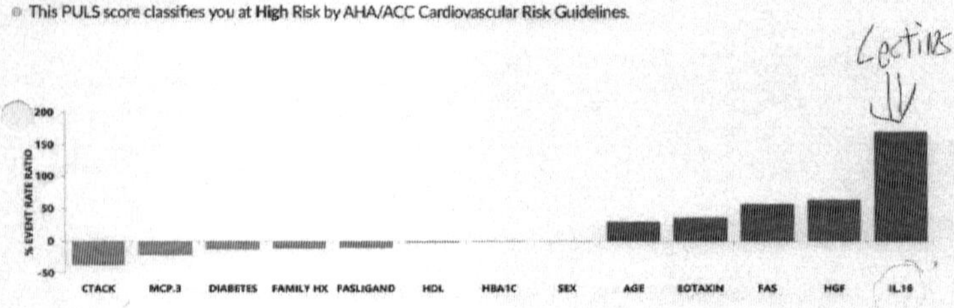

Decreased event ratio Increased event ratio

GRAPH

The size and location of each bar on the Protein Biomarker Graph indicates the relative impact of each biomarker in the formation & progression of cardiac lesions. The chart is read from right to left. Red bars above the zero line indicate factors that increase the probability of experiencing an Acute Coronary Syndrome (ACS). Green bars below the zero line indicate factors that decrease your probability of experiencing an ACS.

PULS CARDIAC TEST						PULS EXPECTED SCORE GAP			
PULS Score (Absolute Risk)	<3.50%	3.50% - 7.49%	15.88 ≥ 7.50%	Expected Score For Age and Sex	3.11	Score Gap (Relative Risk)	<5 Times	5.11 ≥5 Times	
AHA/ACC Guidelines Class	High	This patient is at high risk and should be treated as such. A low threshold for additional testing should be applied to this patient to better define the clinical picture and treatment plan. Aggressive lifestyle modification, supplements, and or medication should be considered. If the clinical situation warrants it, and the patient is not currently under the care of a cardiologist, referral to a cardiologist might be warranted.							

METHODOLOGY: Chemiluminescent Immunoassay and Photometry

Performing Laboratory: GD Biosciences, Inc. Irvine, CA - CLIA#05D2020794 - Lab Director: Douglas S. Harrington, M.D., FASPC, FCAP DCO-021-001 11/06/14

PULS CARDIAC TEST

Doctor Steven Gundry MD
has requested this report for
Meine, David
10/12/18 1027 PST

PATIENT INFORMATION		SPECIMEN INFORMATION	PRACTITIONER INFORMATION
Name Meine, David		Collection Date/Time 10/08/18 1030 PST	Name Gundry, Steven
Age 61	Sex M	Received Date/Time 10/09/18 1000 PST	Client ID 2224 International Heart & Lung
Fasting Status Y	DOB 12/10/1956	Report Date/Time 10/12/18 1027 PST	Address 555 E Tachevah Dr, 3 W103 Palm Springs, CA 92262
Accession ID 27588		Report Status Final	

Patient Acute Coronary Syndrome (ACS) Profile is Elevated

PULS Score: 10.38%

Normal < 3.50% | Borderline 3.50% - 7.49% | Elevated ≥ 7.50%

Expected Score: 2.96%

TEST INTERPRETATION:

- Your PULS score indicates that **10.38%** (Absolute Risk) of individuals of your age, sex, and score had a cardiac event within a 5 year time period. Your expected score of **2.96%** is where you should be according to your current age and sex.
- Your PULS score indicates that you are **3.51** times (Relative Risk) more likely to experience an ACS (heart attack) than would be expected for your age and sex.
- This PULS score classifies you at **High** Risk by AHA/ACC Cardiovascular Risk Guidelines.

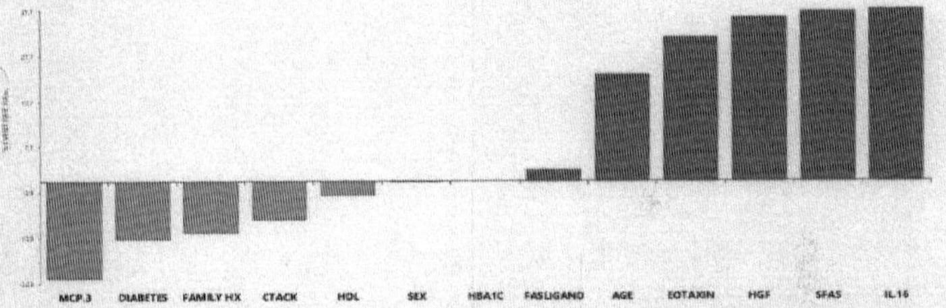

GRAPH

The size and location of each bar on the Protein Biomarker Graph indicates the relative impact of each biomarker in the formation & progression of cardiac lesions. The chart is read from right to left. Red bars above the zero line indicate factors that increase the probability of experiencing an Acute Coronary Syndrome (ACS). Green bars below the zero line indicate factors that decrease your probability of experiencing an ACS.

PULS CARDIAC TEST						PULS EXPECTED SCORE GAP		
PULS Score (Absolute Risk)	< 3.50%	3.50% - 7.49%	10.38 ≥ 7.50%	Expected Score For Age and Sex	2.96	Score Gap (Relative Risk)	3.51 < 5 Times	≥ 5 Times
AHA/ACC Guidelines Class	High	This patient is at high risk and should be treated as such. A low threshold for additional testing should be applied to this patient to better define the clinical picture and treatment plan. Aggressive lifestyle modification, supplements, and or medication should be considered. If the clinical situation warrants it, and the patient is not currently under the care of a cardiologist, referral to a cardiologist might be warranted.						

METHODOLOGY: Chemiluminescent Immunoassay and Photometry

Performing Laboratory: GD Biosciences, Inc. Irvine, CA - CLIA#05D2020794 - Lab Director: Douglas S. Harrington, M.D., FASPC, FCAP

9. Quest Diagnostics Report:

Quest Diagnostics → ClevelandHeartLab® *Know your risk.*

Report Status: Final
MEINE, DAVID

Patient Information	Specimen Information	Client Information
MEINE, DAVID DOB: 12/10/1956 AGE: 62 Gender: Male Fasting: Fasting Phone: Patient ID:	Order ID: 1933801918 Requisition: 1933801918 Collected: 12/03/2019, 00:01 AM Received: 12/04/2019, 3:20 PM Reported: 12/09/2019, 11:28 AM	STEVEN R. GUNDRY, M.D. 14429 INTERNATIONAL HEART AND LUNG INSTITUTE 555 EAST TACHEVAH DRIVE SUITE 3W-103 PALM SPRINGS, CA 92262

Cardiometabolic Report

Test Name	Current: Result & Relative Risk		Reference Range/Relative Risk Categories				Historical: Result & Relative Risk	
	Optimal	Non-Optimal	Optimal	Moderate	High	Units	//	//
INFLAMMATION								
ADMA (Asymmetric dimethylarginine)[1]	91		<100	100-123	>123	ng/mL		
SDMA (Symmetric dimethylarginine)	93			73-135		ng/mL		
OxLDL		64	<60	60-69	≥70	U/L		
LIPIDS								
Apolipoproteins								
Lipoprotein (a)	<10		<75	75-125	>125	nmol/L		
Lipoprotein Subfractions								
sdLDL	35.3		<50.0	N/A	≥50.0	mg/dL		
METABOLIC								
TMAO (Trimethylamine N-oxide)[2]	3.0		<6.2	6.2-9.9	≥10.0	uM		
HYPERTENSION/HEART FAILURE								
Galectin-3	10.5		<17.9	17.9-25.9	>25.9	ng/mL		

UND = UNDETECTABLE INC = INCOMPUTABLE

4myheart Diet & Exercise Coaching Program: Need help achieving and maintaining an optimal weight? Managing stress? Trying to improve physical fitness levels? The 4myheart program provides support and personalized lifestyle guidance to help improve heart health. Please talk to your provider, visit 4myheart.com or call 1-800-432-7889 opt 2 to learn more.

Medical Information For Healthcare Providers: If you have any questions about any of the tests in our Cardiometabolic Report, please call Cleveland HeartLab Client Services at 866.358.9828, option 1 to arrange a consult with our clinical education team.

CLIENT SERVICES: 866.358.9828, Option 1 ORDER ID: 1933801918 Medical Director: Bill G. Richendollar, MD
Cleveland HeartLab, Inc. | 6701 Carnegie Ave. Suite 500 | Cleveland, OH 44103 | p 866-358-9828 | CLIA#36D1032987 | CAP#7190119
Quest, Quest Diagnostics, the associated logo and all associated Quest Diagnostics marks are the trademarks of Quest Diagnostics. Page 1 of 4

10. Supplements Page #2, with Dr. Gundry's Additions:

Supplements

Name: David

Date: ~~12/5/18~~ 1/29/2020

	Acetyl-L-Carnitine 250-500 mg/day
	Alpha Lipoic Acid (sustained release if you can find it) 300 mg/day
	Baby Aspirin once/day
	Biotin 5000 mg/day
	Borage oil 2,000 mg/ am & pm
	Curcumin
	Cholest-off two tablets twice/day (absorbs/blocks cholesterol) (at Costco)
	Chromium Picolinate 200-400 mcg/day
X	Cinnamon ¼ to ½ tsp/day – Cinsulin 1 twice a day (at Costco)
	Co-enzyme Q-10 100 mg/day
	DHEA 25 mg
X	Fish oil DHA 1,000 mg/day
	Flax Seed Oil 1,000 mg/day
	5-HTP
X	Ginkgo Biloba 120 mg 2 a day
	Grape seed Extract 100 mg/day
	Green Tea Extract 200-500 mg/day
	Hawthorne 250-500 mg/day (Dr.'s Best/Clarks)
	Huperzine A 100 mcg/day
	Kaolic Garlic Heart Formula 106 two twice/day
	L-Reuteri (5 billion)
	Magnesium (potassium asporatate) 400 mg/day
X	Methyl B12 5,000 mcg Kirkland (Costco) sublingual 1 under tongue a day
X	Methylfolate 1,000 mcg/day 1 a day
	Milk Thistle
	Modified Citrus Pectin
	N-Acetyl-Cysteine (better known as NAC) 250-500 mg/day
	Niacin 500 mg
	No Flush Niacin 500 mg (extended release)
	Slo-Niacin 500 mg at night with 325 mg Tylenol *After two weeks increase to 1,000 mg
(X)	Pregnenolone 50/100 mg 50mg (1)
	Pycnogenol 25-50 mg/day
	Quercetin 500 mg 2/day
	Red Yeast Rice Extract 600 to 1,200 mg/day
	Relora
	Rhodiola 100-500 mg/day
	Selenium 200 mcg/day
	Spirulina
X	Tumeric Extract (curcumin) (With BioPerine) ~~900mg twice/day (Vitacost.com)~~ You Theory @ Costco 3 a day
X	Vit-C 1000 mg twice/day
(X)	Vit-D3 5,000 IU, [illegible]/day ~~10,000~~ IUs daily 15,000
	Vit-K2
	Schiff Digestive Advantage (Probiotic)
X	Pau D'Arco 500mg 2 a day
X	Brassica Tea 2 cups daily (baltersftcc.com)
X	Vital Reds, Total Restore, Primal Plants, Lectin Shield 6 months

11. Dexa Body Scan Report:

Dexa Body

2046 Murray Holladay Road
Suite 201
Holladay, Utah 84117
(801) 274-3392

David Meine **Measured: 06/15/2020**

Age: 63.5 **Birth Date:** 12/10/1956
Gender: Male **Height:** 72.0 in.
Baseline Date: (none) **Weight:** 198.0 lbs.

SUMMARY LEVEL RESULTS

Total Body Composition

Measured Date	Total Body Fat	Total Tissue Mass (lbs)	Fat Tissue (lbs)	Lean Tissue (lbs)	Bone Mineral Content (BMC)
06/15/2020	27.5%	198.2 lbs	52.5 lbs	138.5 lbs	7.1 lbs
09/13/2018	25.7%	197.8 lbs	48.9 lbs	141.6 lbs	7.4 lbs
06/12/2018	26.5%	198.9 lbs	50.7 lbs	140.8 lbs	7.4 lbs

Total Body Tissue Quantitation

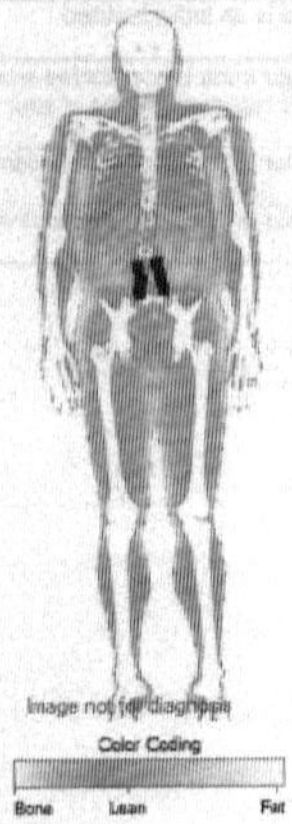

Ideal Body Fat Percentage

This table provides target body fat percentages based on American Council on Exercise recommendations.

Description	Men	Women
Essential Fat	2 - 5%	10 - 13%
Athletes	6 - 13%	14 - 20%
Fitness	14 - 17%	21 - 24%
Average	18 - 24%	25 - 31%
Above Average	25% +	32% +

Regional Composition

The table below divides your body into 5 key regions and provides the composition breakdown for each. Dexa Body will track these regions over time to chart individual progress.

Region	Total Region Fat %	Total Mass (lbs)	Fat Tissue (lbs)	Lean Tissue (lbs)	Bone Mineral Content (BMC)
Arms	23.0%	23.9 lbs	5.5 lbs	17.3 lbs	1.2 lbs
Legs	17.2%	61.6 lbs	10.8 lbs	48.3 lbs	2.8 lbs
Trunk	33.8%	101.2 lbs	34.2 lbs	65.0 lbs	2.0 lbs
Android	38.8%	15.1 lbs	5.8 lbs	9.1 lbs	0.1 lbs
Gynoid	22.1%	28.6 lbs	6.3 lbs	21.6 lbs	0.7 lbs

Page: 1 of 10

Dexa Body

2046 Murray Holladay Road
Suite 201
Holladay, Utah 84117
(801) 274-3392

Client	Sex	Facility	Birth Date	Height	Weight	Measured
David Maine	Male	Utah Office	12/10/1956	72.0 in.	198.0 lbs.	09/15/2020

METABOLIC & MUSCLE DISTRIBUTION REPORT

RESTING METABOLIC RATE (RMR)		
Test Date 09/15/2020	1,785 cal/day	This is a nutritional baseline indicating the number of calories you need to intake to sustain lean tissue. Depending on your goals, you will need a caloric deficit or surplus. Dexa Body offers a comprehensive RMR test which offers an in depth calculation of your total body caloric requirements.

RELATIVE SKELETAL MUSCLE INDEX (RSMI)		
Test Date 09/15/2020	8.86 kg/m²	RSMI represents the relative amount of muscle in the arms and legs. Sarcopenia is the degenerative loss of skeletal mass (0.5 - 1% loss per year after the age of 25), quality, and strength associated with aging. Men should have an RSMI greater than 7.26, and women should be greater than 5.45.

LEAN MASS RATIOS		
Lean mass ratios provide a quick snapshot of how lean tissue is distributed in our bodies. This is an individualized approach to understanding lean tissue distribution relative to your total body composition.		
Trunk	69.6%	This metric indicates what percentage of the total tissue in your trunk is considered lean tissue. The trunk includes the area spanning from your pelvic region to the top of your neck, not including your arms.
Legs	80.6%	This metric indicates what percentage of the total tissue in your legs is considered lean tissue.
Arms	74.8%	This metric indicates what percentage of the total tissue in your arms is considered lean tissue.

Page: 2 of 10

Dexa Body

2046 Murray Holladay Road
Suite 201
Holladay, Utah 84117
(801) 274-3392

FAT DISTRIBUTION REPORT

Abdomen Composition

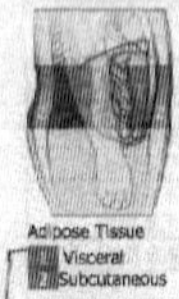

The Android region is that of the abdomen, and often the body type with increased fat in this area is described as "apple shaped." The Gynoid region is that around the hips and thighs and often the body type with increased fat in this area is described as "pear shaped." Understanding where fat is stored on the body is recognized as an important predictor of the potential health risks of obesity. The A/G ratio compares Android fat to Gynoid fat. The ideal ratio is less than **1.0** for optimal fat distribution.

Dexa Body estimates the VAT (Visceral Adipose Tissue) content within the android region, VAT is a specific type of fat that is associated with several types of metabolic diseases such as obesity, metabolic syndrome, and type 2 diabetes. Dexa Body results have been validated for adults between ages 18-90, and with a BMI in the range of 18.5-40.

Total

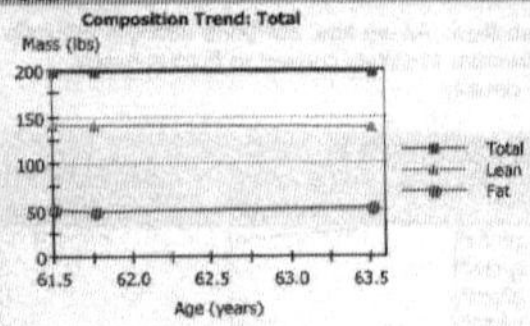

Date	Age	Total Mass (lbs)	Lean Mass (lbs)	Fat Mass (lbs)
06/12/2018	61.5	198.9	140.8	50.7
09/13/2018	61.7	197.8	141.6	48.9
06/15/2020	63.5	198.2	138.5	52.5

Android / Gynoid

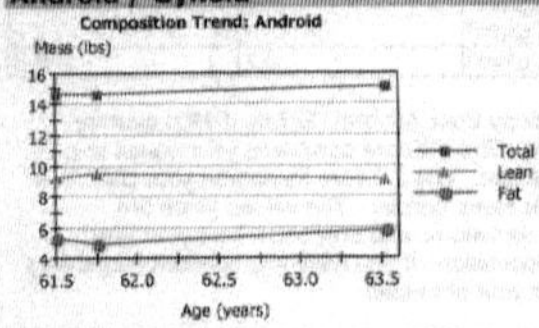

Date	Age	Android Mass (lbs)	Android Lean (lbs)	Android Fat (lbs)	Android %Fat	Gynoid %Fat	A/G Ratio
06/12/2018	61.5	14.7	9.3	5.3	36.6	22.2	1.65
09/13/2018	61.7	14.7	9.5	5.0	34.6	22.1	1.56
06/15/2020	63.5	15.1	9.1	5.8	39.0	22.6	1.73

Visceral Adipose Tissue (VAT)

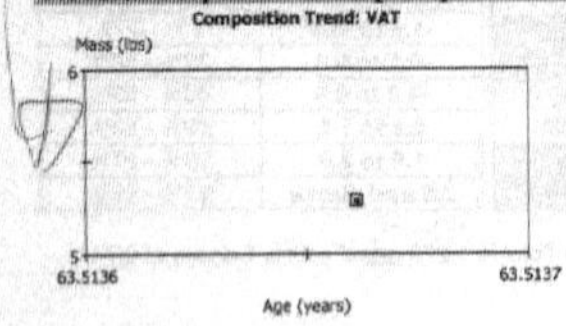

Date	Age	Fat Mass (lbs)	Volume (in³)
06/15/2020	63.5	5.29	155.34

Less than 1 lb

Page: 3 of 10

Dexa Body

2046 Murray Holladay Road
Suite 201
Holladay, Utah 84117
(801) 274-3392

Client	Sex	Facility	Birth Date	Height	Weight	Measured
David Meine	Male	Utah Office	12/10/1956	72.0 in.	198.0 lbs.	06/15/2020

MUSCLE BALANCE REPORT

The table below regionalizes your arms and legs to assess muscle symmetry. Arms will often have tissue imbalances up to 0.5 lbs, while legs will have tissue imbalances up to 1.5 lbs. Dexa Body looks at movement efficiency, and having a balanced body composition improves overall physical capability, especially with functional movements.

Region	% Fat	Total Mass	Fat Mass	Lean Mass	BMC
Right Arm	23.2%	12.5 lbs	2.9 lbs	9.0 lbs	0.6 lbs
Left Arm	22.8%	11.4 lbs	2.6 lbs	8.2 lbs	0.6 lbs
Arms Total	**23.0%**	**23.9 lbs**	**5.6 lbs**	**17.3 lbs**	**1.2 lbs**
Right Leg	17.2%	31.0 lbs	5.3 lbs	24.3 lbs	1.4 lbs
Left Leg	17.2%	30.6 lbs	5.3 lbs	23.9 lbs	1.4 lbs
Legs Total	**17.2%**	**61.6 lbs**	**10.6 lbs**	**48.3 lbs**	**2.8 lbs**

BONE REPORT

Bone density is a critical component of our overall health and physical capabilities. As we age, our bone strength naturally deteriorates through a process called fibrosis. Fibrosis causes our bone structure to slowly convert to fibrous tissue. Weight-bearing exercises that stress our skeletal tissue can increase bone density.

Total Body Bone Density

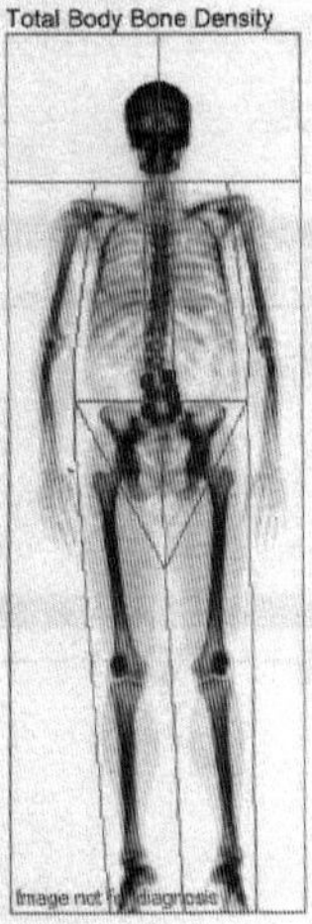

Bone Density: USA (Combined NHANES/Lunar)

Region	BMD	Young Adult T-Score	Age Matched Z-Score
Head	2.183 g/cm²	-	-
Arms	0.874 g/cm²	-	-
Legs	1.463 g/cm²	-	-
Trunk	1.086 g/cm²	-	-
Ribs	0.962 g/cm²	-	-
Spine	1.275 g/cm²	-	-
Pelvis	1.094 g/cm²	-	-
Total	1.272 g/cm²	0.7	0.5

The chart above provides a Total Body Bone Mineral Density (BMD) quantity along with a T-Score and a Z-Score. The T-Score compares your bones to a healthy 30-year old adult of your gender. The Z-Score compares your BMD to a person at your same age and of the same gender. The values given are measured in units called standard deviations, and they show how your BMD compares to the given reference population. If you have any concerns regarding these numbers, you should contact your physician.

T-Score	Result
-1 and above	Normal
-1.0 to -2.5	Potential Osteopenia
-2.5 and below	Potential Osteoporosis

Z Score	% Population (Greater Than)
-1.5 to -0.5	7% - 30%
-0.5 to 0.0	30% - 50%
-0.0 to 0.5	50% - 69%
0.5 to 1.5	69% - 93%
1.5 to 2.0	93% - 97%
2.0 and above	97% - 99%

The BMD measured at Total Body Total is 1.272 g/cm² with a T-score of 0.7 is normal. Fracture risk is low.

Page: 4 of 10

Dexa Body

2046 Murray Holladay Road
Suite 201
Holladay, Utah 84117
(801) 274-3392

Client	Sex	Facility	Birth Date	Height	Weight	Measured
David Meine	Male	Utah Office	12/10/1956	72.0 in.	198.0 lbs.	06/15/2020

REGIONAL FAT TISSUE REPORT

The following graphs display how fat tissue in different regions of your body have changed over time. These graphs show how the different regions in your body have responded to your training and/or nutrition program. Each individual will gain and lose fat differently. Dexa Body will continue to track and report on each of these regions in follow up scans.

Arms

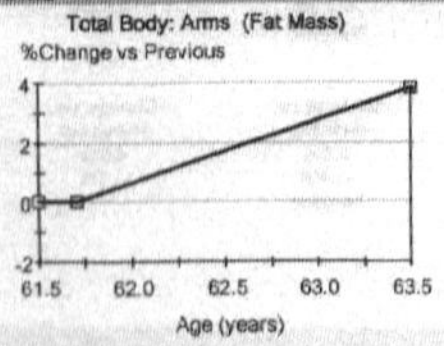

Measured Date	Region Fat Totals	Change vs. Baseline	Change vs. Previous
06/15/2020	5.5 lbs	0.2 lbs	0.2 lbs
09/13/2018	5.3 lbs	0.0 lbs	0.0 lbs
06/12/2018	5.3 lbs	baseline	-

Measured Date	Region Fat Percent	Change vs. Baseline	Change vs. Previous
06/15/2020	23.0%	1.4%	2.3%
09/13/2018	20.7%	-0.9%	-0.9%
06/12/2018	21.6%	baseline	-

Legs

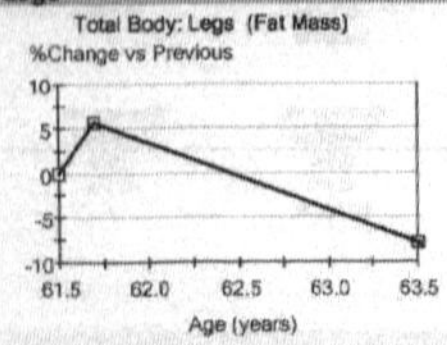

Measured Date	Region Fat Totals	Change vs. Baseline	Change vs. Previous
06/15/2020	10.6 lbs	-0.3 lbs	-0.9 lbs
09/13/2018	11.5 lbs	0.6 lbs	0.6 lbs
06/12/2018	10.9 lbs	baseline	-

Measured Date	Region Fat Percent	Change vs. Baseline	Change vs. Previous
06/15/2020	17.2%	0.2%	-1.1%
09/13/2018	18.3%	1.3%	1.3%
06/12/2018	17.0%	baseline	-

Trunk

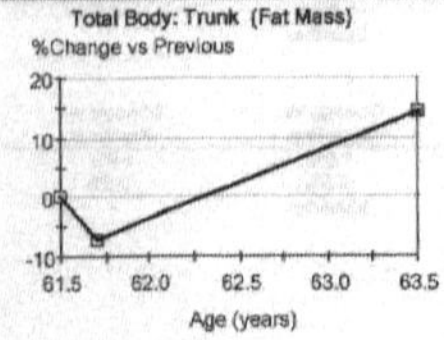

Measured Date	Region Fat Totals	Change vs. Baseline	Change vs. Previous
06/15/2020	34.2 lbs	2.0 lbs	4.3 lbs
09/13/2018	29.9 lbs	-2.3 lbs	-2.3 lbs
06/12/2018	32.2 lbs	baseline	-

Measured Date	Region Fat Percent	Change vs. Baseline	Change vs. Previous
06/15/2020	33.8%	1.1%	3.3%
09/13/2018	30.5%	-2.2%	-2.2%
06/12/2018	32.7%	baseline	-

Page: 5 of 10

Dexa Body

2046 Murray Holladay Road
Suite 201
Holladay, Utah 84117
(801) 274-3392

Client	Sex	Facility	Birth Date	Height	Weight	Measured
David Meine	Male	Utah Office	12/10/1956	72.0 in.	198.0 lbs.	06/15/2020

REGIONAL FAT TISSUE REPORT (Continued)

Android

Total Body: Android (Fat Mass)
%Change vs Previous

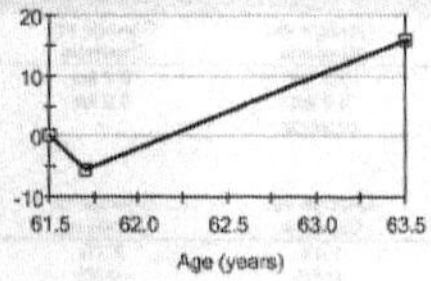

Measured Date	Region Fat Totals	Change vs. Baseline	Change vs. Previous
06/15/2020	5.8 lbs	0.6 lbs	0.8 lbs
09/13/2018	5.0 lbs	-0.3 lbs	-0.3 lbs
06/12/2018	5.3 lbs	baseline	-

Measured Date	Region Fat Percent	Change vs. Baseline	Change vs. Previous
06/15/2020	38.8%	2.5%	4.6%
09/13/2018	34.2%	-2.1%	-2.1%
06/12/2018	36.3%	baseline	-

Gynoid

Total Body: Gynoid (Fat Mass)
%Change vs Previous

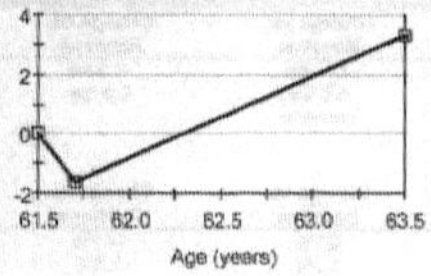

Measured Date	Region Fat Totals	Change vs. Baseline	Change vs. Previous
06/15/2020	6.3 lbs	0.1 lbs	0.2 lbs
09/13/2018	6.1 lbs	-0.1 lbs	-0.1 lbs
06/12/2018	6.2 lbs	baseline	-

Measured Date	Region Fat Percent	Change vs. Baseline	Change vs. Previous
06/15/2020	22.1%	0.5%	0.6%
09/13/2018	21.5%	-0.1%	-0.1%
06/12/2018	21.6%	baseline	-

Total

Total Body: Total (Fat Mass)
%Change vs Previous

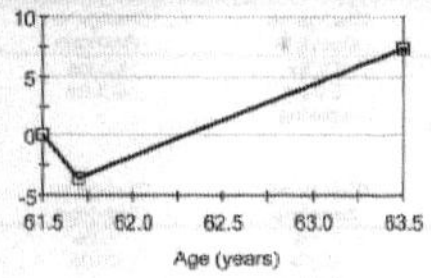

Measured Date	Region Fat Totals	Change vs. Baseline	Change vs. Previous
06/15/2020	52.5 lbs	1.8 lbs	3.6 lbs
09/13/2018	48.9 lbs	-1.8 lbs	-1.8 lbs
06/12/2018	50.7 lbs	baseline	-

Measured Date	Region Fat Percent	Change vs. Baseline	Change vs. Previous
06/15/2020	26.5%	1.0%	1.8%
09/13/2018	24.7%	-0.8%	-0.8%
06/12/2018	25.6%	baseline	-

Page: 6 of 10

Dexa Body

2046 Murray Holladay Road
Suite 201
Holladay, Utah 84117
(801) 274-3392

Client	Sex	Facility	Birth Date	Height	Weight	Measured
David Meine	Male	Utah Office	12/10/1956	72.0 in.	198.0 lbs.	06/15/2020

REGIONAL LEAN TISSUE REPORT

The following graphs display how lean tissue in different regions of your body have changed over time. These graphs show how the different regions in your body have responded to your training and/or nutrition program. Each individual will gain and lose lean mass differently. Dexa Body will continue to track and report on each of these regions in follow up scans.

Arms

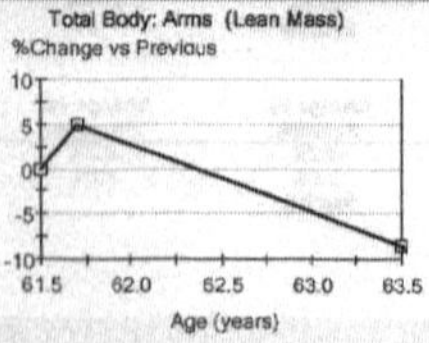

Measured Date	Region Lean Totals	Change vs. Baseline	Change vs. Previous
06/15/2020	17.3 lbs	-0.7 lbs	-1.6 lbs
09/13/2018	18.9 lbs	0.9 lbs	0.9 lbs
06/12/2018	18.0 lbs	baseline	-

Measured Date	Region Lean Percent	Change vs. Baseline	Change vs. Previous
06/15/2020	72.2%	-3.9%	-8.5%
09/13/2018	74.6%	5.0%	5.0%
06/12/2018	73.5%	baseline	-

Legs

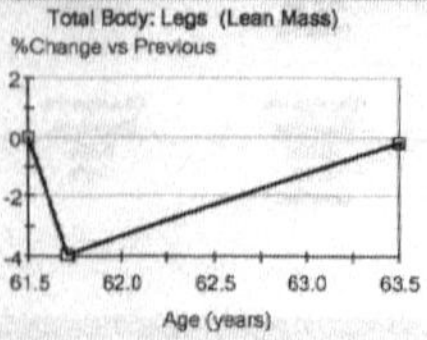

Measured Date	Region Lean Totals	Change vs. Baseline	Change vs. Previous
06/15/2020	48.3 lbs	-2.1 lbs	-0.1 lbs
09/13/2018	48.4 lbs	-2.0 lbs	-2.0 lbs
06/12/2018	50.4 lbs	baseline	-

Measured Date	Region Lean Percent	Change vs. Baseline	Change vs. Previous
06/15/2020	78.3%	-4.2%	-0.2%
09/13/2018	77.0%	-4.0%	-4.0%
06/12/2018	78.4%	baseline	-

Trunk

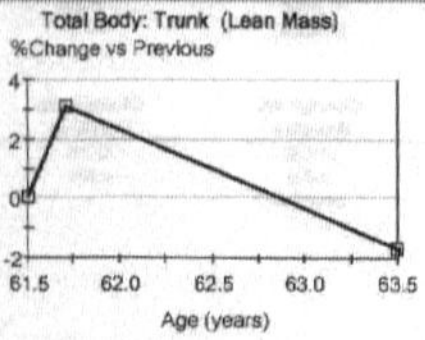

Measured Date	Region Lean Totals	Change vs. Baseline	Change vs. Previous
06/15/2020	65.0 lbs	0.9 lbs	-1.1 lbs
09/13/2018	66.1 lbs	2.0 lbs	2.0 lbs
06/12/2018	64.1 lbs	baseline	-

Measured Date	Region Lean Percent	Change vs. Baseline	Change vs. Previous
06/15/2020	64.3%	1.4%	-1.7%
09/13/2018	67.4%	3.1%	3.1%
06/12/2018	65.2%	baseline	-

Page: 7 of 10

Dexa Body

2046 Murray Holladay Road
Suite 201
Holladay, Utah 84117
(801) 274-3392

Client	Sex	Facility	Birth Date	Height	Weight	Measured
David Meine	Male	Utah Office	12/10/1956	72.0 in.	198.0 lbs.	06/15/2020

REGIONAL LEAN TISSUE REPORT (Continued)

Android

Total Body: Android (Lean Mass)
%Change vs Previous

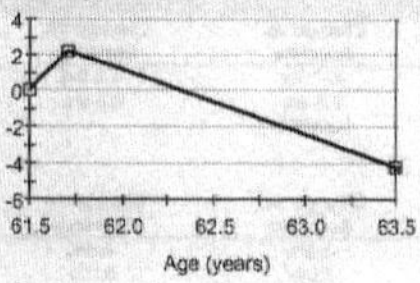

Measured Date	Region Lean Totals	Change vs. Baseline	Change vs. Previous
06/15/2020	9.1 lbs	-0.2 lbs	-0.4 lbs
09/13/2018	9.5 lbs	0.2 lbs	0.2 lbs
06/12/2018	9.3 lbs	baseline	-

Measured Date	Region Lean Percent	Change vs. Baseline	Change vs. Previous
06/15/2020	60.6%	-2.2%	-4.2%
09/13/2018	64.8%	2.2%	2.2%
06/12/2018	62.9%	baseline	-

Gynoid

Total Body: Gynoid (Lean Mass)
%Change vs Previous

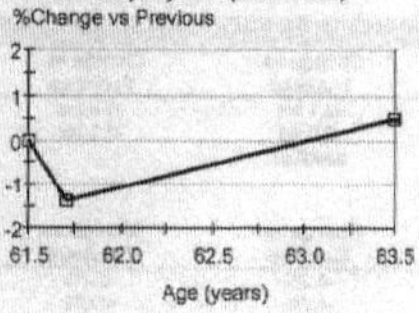

Measured Date	Region Lean Totals	Change vs. Baseline	Change vs. Previous
06/15/2020	21.6 lbs	-0.2 lbs	0.1 lbs
09/13/2018	21.5 lbs	-0.3 lbs	-0.3 lbs
06/12/2018	21.8 lbs	baseline	-

Measured Date	Region Lean Percent	Change vs. Baseline	Change vs. Previous
06/15/2020	69.9%	-0.9%	0.5%
09/13/2018	71.8%	-1.4%	-1.4%
06/12/2018	70.8%	baseline	-

Total

Total Body: Total (Lean Mass)
%Change vs Previous

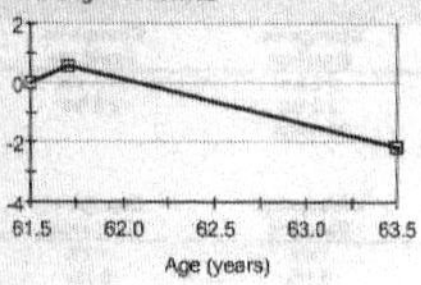

Measured Date	Region Lean Totals	Change vs. Baseline	Change vs. Previous
06/15/2020	138.5 lbs	-2.3 lbs	-3.1 lbs
09/13/2018	141.6 lbs	0.8 lbs	0.8 lbs
06/12/2018	140.8 lbs	baseline	-

Measured Date	Region Lean Percent	Change vs. Baseline	Change vs. Previous
06/15/2020	69.9%	-1.8%	-2.2%
09/13/2018	71.6%	0.6%	0.6%
06/12/2018	70.8%	baseline	-

Page: 8 of 10

Dexa Body

2046 Murray Holladay Road
Suite 201
Holladay, Utah 84117
(801) 274-3392

Client	Sex	Facility	Birth Date	Height	Weight	Measured
David Meine	Male	Utah Office	12/10/1956	72.0 in.	198.0 lbs.	06/15/2020

REGIONAL BONE REPORT

Arms

Total Body: Arms (BMD)

%Change vs Baseline

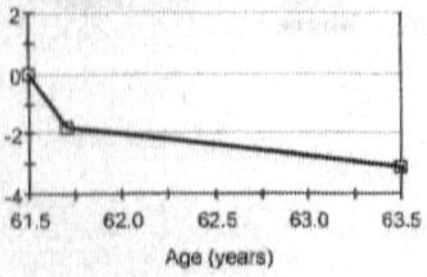

Measured Date	BMD	Change vs. Baseline	Change vs. Previous
06/15/2020	0.874 g/cm²	5 cm²	-11 cm²
09/13/2018	0.886 g/cm²	16 cm²	16 cm²
06/12/2018	0.902 g/cm²	baseline	-

Legs

Total Body: Legs (BMD)

%Change vs Baseline

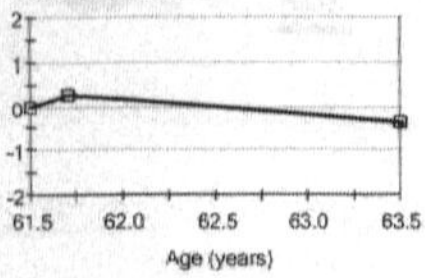

Measured Date	BMD	Change vs. Baseline	Change vs. Previous
06/15/2020	1.463 g/cm²	-32 cm²	-35 cm²
09/13/2018	1.472 g/cm²	3 cm²	3 cm²
06/12/2018	1.468 g/cm²	baseline	-

Trunk

Total Body: Trunk (BMD)

%Change vs Baseline

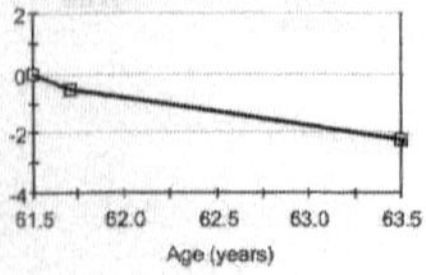

Measured Date	BMD	Change vs. Baseline	Change vs. Previous
06/15/2020	1.463 g/cm²	-40 cm²	-13 cm²
09/13/2018	1.472 g/cm²	-27 cm²	-27 cm²
06/12/2018	1.468 g/cm²	baseline	-

Page: 9 of 10

Dexa Body

2046 Murray Holladay Road
Suite 201
Holladay, Utah 84117
(801) 274-3392

Client	Sex	Facility	Birth Date	Height	Weight	Measured
David Meine	Male	Utah Office	12/10/1956	72.0 in.	198.0 lbs.	06/15/2020

REGIONAL BONE REPORT (Continued)

Ribs

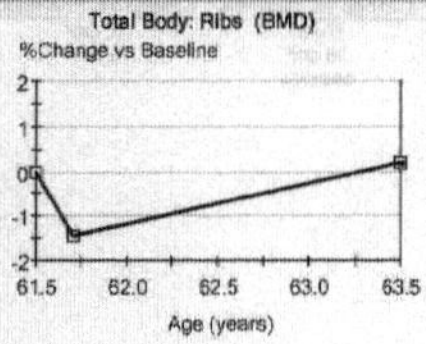

Measured Date	BMD	Change vs. Baseline	Change vs. Previous
06/15/2020	0.962 g/cm²	20 cm²	9 cm²
09/13/2018	0.946 g/cm²	11 cm²	11 cm²
06/12/2018	0.960 g/cm²	baseline	-

Spine

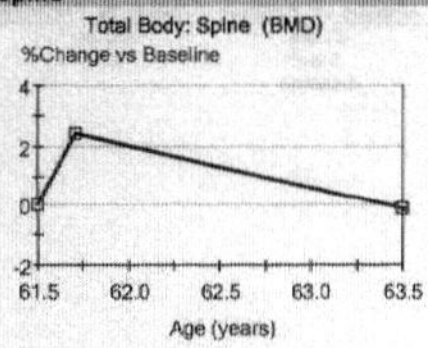

Measured Date	BMD	Change vs. Baseline	Change vs. Previous
06/15/2020	1.275 g/cm²	-9 cm²	-4 cm²
09/13/2018	1.307 g/cm²	-5 cm²	-5 cm²
06/12/2018	1.276 g/cm²	baseline	-

Pelvis

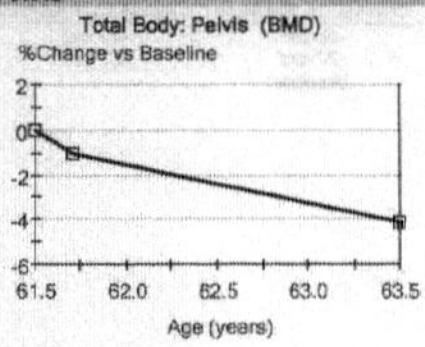

Measured Date	BMD	Change vs. Baseline	Change vs. Previous
06/15/2020	1.094 g/cm²	-50 cm²	-18 cm²
09/13/2018	1.129 g/cm²	-32 cm²	-32 cm²
06/12/2018	1.141 g/cm²	baseline	-

Note: Dexa Body is not a medical facility, nor do we represent the views of any medical practitioner. The data provided in this report is for informational purposes only and is not meant to be used for any type of medical diagnoses. If you have any concerns regarding the data or metrics in this report, please consult with your physician.

Page: 10 of 10